T5-CCW-116

# I Have Fibromyalgia / Chronic Fatigue Syndrome, but it Doesn't Have Me! A Memoir

**SIX STEPS FOR REVERSING FMS/CFS**

Chantal K. Hoey-Sanders

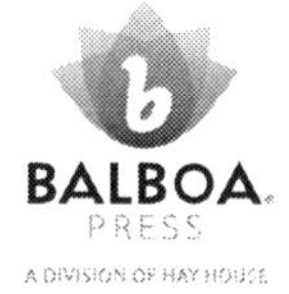

*Disclaimer: This book contains advice and information relating to healthcare. It is not intended to replace medical advice. Rather, it should be used to supplement rather than replace regular care by your doctor. It is recommended that you seek your physician's advice before embarking on any medical treatment or program. The author has made every attempt to be accurate in conveying information about fibromyalgia/chronic fatigue syndrome in this book (as of the date of publication). The publisher, the editor, and the author assume no responsibility for errors, inaccuracies, omissions, or any inconsistencies herein. This book is not intended as a diagnostic tool. Please consult medical professionals for your personal health problems. Internet addresses given in this book were accurate at the time it went to press.*

*Balboa Press books may be ordered through booksellers or by contacting:*

*Balboa Press*
*A Division of Hay House*
*1663 Liberty Drive*
*Bloomington, IN 47403*
*www.balboapress.com*
*1-(877) 407-4847*

*Because of the dynamic nature of the Internet, any Web addresses or links contained in this book may have changed since publication and may no longer be valid. The views expressed in this work are solely those of the author and do not necessarily reflect the views of the publisher, and the publisher hereby disclaims any responsibility for them.*

*The author of this book does not dispense medical advice or prescribe the use of any technique as a form of treatment for physical, emotional, or medical problems without the advice of a physician, either directly or indirectly. The intent of the author is only to offer information of a general nature to help you in your quest for emotional and spiritual well-being. In the event you use any of the information in this book for yourself, which is your constitutional right, the author and the publisher assume no responsibility for your actions.*



*ISBN: 978-1-4525-0147-5 (sc)*
*ISBN: 978-1-4525-0149-9 (dj)*
*ISBN: 978-1-4525-0148-2 (e)*

*Library of Congress Control Number: 2010917693*

*Printed in the United States of America*
*Balboa Press rev. date: 04/11/2011*

For Josh and Alexander:
You are the reason.
Huge heart hugs *always.*

# Contents

# Acknowledgments

Eight years in the making, this book would not be in existence if it weren't for the following people:

Dr. R. Paul St. Amand, founder of the Guaifenesin Protocol
Thank you for having the courage to stick with your convictions and share with the world this amazing protocol.

Claudia Craig Marek, author and GuaiGroup leader
Thank you for your dedication, encouragement, and support throughout my process of following the Guaifenesin Protocol.

Anne Louise, Char, Cris, Gretchen, and Jan the GuaiGroup Administrators
Thank you for your dedication.

Thaddeus Srutwa, MD, acupuncturist, confidante, and friend who rescued me when I was drowning, believed in me, and introduced me to the Guaifenesin Protocol
I am forever grateful.

Almeda Russell, forty years my senior and six months ahead of me on the protocol
Thank you for your hours of encouragement, friendship, and telephone support.

Kim Dake, my friend, who faithfully picked me up every Monday morning and took me grocery shopping

I needed your friendship, patience, and kindness more than you will ever know.

Christina Anderson, "Sistermoon," fellow fibromyalgic
You are my Light.

Robert Picard, family friend and meditation mentor
*Namaste.*

Ann Mitchell, my brilliant high school English teacher, who spent countless hours editing my work
You shine.

Kris Bruinsma and Harriett Jones, my faithful fibro-readers
Thank you for the endless hours you spent reviewing my work.

I am also very grateful to my family.
They say it takes a whole village to raise a child. Well, it also takes a whole village to recover from fibromyalgia/chronic fatigue syndrome. A special thanks to:

Robert Crego, my adopted Grandfather and beacon, who always provides unconditional support; Hilda Raus, my now deceased Grandmother who taught me how to crochet and sew; Katie Hoey, my mom, who loves me unconditionally, supports me, and never doubted that I would one day become a mother; Charles J. Hoey, my father, who has confidence in me when I don't; Michelle Hoey-Heath, my sister, who, as she puts it "carted my ass around town" for years when I was too sick to drive; Nicole Hoey, my sister, who insisted I try acupuncture; Nikolaus Sanders, my step-son, who played endless hours of *Pooh* memory with me in the hope that I would one day regain my short-term memory; Jill Sanders, my mother-in-law, who flew with me to Mayo Clinic for further testing; Neil Sanders, my now deceased father-in-law, who introduced me to the power of eating the way that is "right for your body"; Josh Sanders, my loyal husband, who has spent thousands of hours waiting in the car, driving me to and from many of my appointments over the years. Words can't express my gratitude and love for you; and Alexander Sanders, Mama's greatest joy—I love you to the moon and back!

# Foreword

In this book, Chantal shares her struggles to come to terms with and triumph over fibromyalgia's effects on her life. She has been through the vicissitudes: beginning with grief and loss and ending with an understanding that she is not her illness.

She tells you how she did it and offers the reader a vision of her duet dance with a non-cooperative foe. She battles the enemy fibromyalgia in her mind, her body, and her spirit. It is difficult not to admire her; the work and willpower she demonstrates are remarkable. She stands on her own two feet despite her difficulties and never gives up for long. She has met her future and learned the protocol that will make her well.

Let's be grateful for people such as Chantal. She's not interested in just saving herself, but in showing her path to others. She hopes to motivate you to join her. Take her lead, read her book, and hold on to her rollercoaster ride to understanding.

R. Paul St. Amand, MD
Associate Clinical Professor of Medicine, Harbor UCLA
September 1, 2010

# Preface

I have been writing this book since I first got sick in 2002.

A year before being officially diagnosed with fibromyalgia, I became gravely ill with a migraine that never went away. It left me completely bedridden and unable to function. I had to take a leave of absence from my job. I couldn't read or write. My fibromyalgia had jumbled my brain. I had reverted back into infancy. I was angry and alone.

As a way to pull myself out of my isolation and to work through my own frustration, anger, and fear, I began to tell my story on a handheld tape recorder to myself. I used this voice-activated recorder in the bathroom on the countertop while soaking in the tub. As pathetic as it sounds, soaking in the tub was my only activity for the day. It was the only time that my muscles could become relaxed and my brain could become clear enough to think. I spent the rest of my day bedridden on a futon mattress on the floor in our living room. I was too fatigued and weak to climb the stairs to our bedroom.

Capturing my story on tape was my therapy; my way to try to make sense of what I was experiencing. I never intended anyone else to ever hear it or to read it. It was my therapy and my therapy alone.

I told my story to myself in isolation for one year, not knowing exactly what was wrong with me until I became officially diagnosed with fibromyalgia/chronic fatigue syndrome in 2003.

Now, newly diagnosed, I thirsted to read stories about others with fibromyalgia/chronic fatigue syndrome. I wanted to hear their stories. I wanted to know them. I wanted reassurance that I would one day become well enough to have my own children and care for them.

Newly disabled, I needed to learn how to apply for disability and how to keep myself from feeling like such a failure. I needed to know what kept others with fibromyalgia going on a daily basis when they were living with such an invisible illness and in so much pain. How did they interact with their families and the outside world? Could I find a way to get well that didn't involve a medicine cabinet filled of narcotics and other pills to bandage my individual symptoms? Was there truly hope for me?

Those are the stories I longed for, but few existed. So, here is my story for you, my story of hope and personal empowerment—how I have been able to turn my struggle into my source of strength. And you can, too!

# A Note to My Readers

My goal in sharing my fibromyalgia/chronic fatigue story with you is to show you that hope is here, even when your world looks grim and you feel completely isolated and out of control. I am living proof of it. I went from *bedridden* to *better*—and you can too.

I hope and believe that by sharing my story, you will find an option to help you step out of your fibromyalgia /chronic fatigue story with a safe and effective reversal for this condition. My intent is not to explain Dr. St. Amand's protocol in great detail; rather, it's to introduce you to it and show you the steps that I took to reverse my fibromyalgia enough so I could lead the life that I greatly desired.

I am still a work-in-progress and very happy with my status. I do need to make clear that this is *not* a cure for fibromyalgia: it is a *reversal.* At this present time, no cure exists. However, we are presently living in a hope-filled time with ongoing research.

I chose to try this treatment option for a couple of different reasons. My first reason for giving the Guaifenesin pronounced [("gwy-FEN-e-sin" or Guai "gwy")] Protocol a chance was that I could relate to the authors. Their story was my story and each page of their book brought tears to my eyes, resonated with me, and gave me encouragement.

I was tired of wasting money on treatments that promised me something and never delivered. I was also fed up with my medicine chest full of poly pharmaceuticals that only bandaged my symptoms, and I wasn't willing to go the narcotics route. The Guaifenesin that is used in the reversal process is a safe and relatively inexpensive medication that is available over the counter. Dr. St. Amand does not profit from its sales.

My second reason for trying the protocol was that I was thoroughly impressed with Dr. St. Amand, who has fibromyalgia himself. He has dedicated more than fifty years of his life to fibromyalgia research and continues to do so with the City of Hope genetic research studies in Duarte, California.

Dr. St. Amand is an inspiration. He has reversed his fibromyalgia and plays tennis every day, teaches, and keeps a full-time medical practice at eighty-two years young! It was the word "tennis" that gripped me when I first read his biography and the fact that he still plays. My tennis days came to a screeching halt in my mid-twenties, thanks to my chronic fatigue. I believe we all deserve and can achieve perfect health.

Enjoy and be well.

*Chantal K. Hoey-Sanders*

# Part 1

## Recognizing Fibromyalgia/Chronic Fatigue Syndrome

# Chapter 1: The First Step: Being Diagnosed

"I can be changed by what happens to me, but I refuse to be reduced by it."

—Maya Angelou

## Living with the Frustration of Fibromyalgia *before* Diagnosis

I am alone. I am naked. I am in the bathtub. I am watching the water rise. I have no idea of how I got here. The water is warm and it is getting higher. I am afraid. I begin to laugh. My laughter fills the room and disguises my fear for an instant. Something is really wrong with me. I sense it, feel it, but I don't know what to do. I can't remember how to turn the water off. I am waiting for the flood.

I am alone. I am in my car. The engine is on, but I'm not moving. I'm confused. Something is very wrong, but I don't know what.

I am alone. I am dressed. I am at the grocery store. I need to get some tomatoes. I look down at my hand and at the plastic bag that I am holding. I start to sweat. I stare at the bag, unable to open it. I am clueless. I am dizzy and nearly faint. What is happening to me, to my body, and to my brain?

I am alone. I am in the kitchen. I smell something so potently foul, I am sure that it is a dead rodent. I call to my husband to come in and have a smell. He smells nothing. The odor is very strong. He smells nothing. I am convinced that something has died in our kitchen, maybe in between the walls.

I am alone. I look into the mirror. I see someone. It's not me. I am trapped in a body that is not my own, with a memory that has failed me.

It's early September, my favorite month of the year, but I am too sick to care.

I am thirty-two years old, newly married, a wife, a stepmother, a high school Spanish teacher with her master's degree. I love to travel and to help others. But, I ask myself, "Who am I?"

I spend the next year with a throbbing daily migraine headache that pierces through my face and eyes. My vision comes and goes. Pain soars throughout my body. One day, I can't move my hands and fingers. The next day, I urinate fifty times within an hour. I can't sleep. I have problems swallowing. I can no longer read or write. My eyes and brain don't allow it. I pray to God that this is not MS.

Every day, this headache is getting worse. My ears are ringing. My eyes can't tolerate any light. The left sides of my face and body are frozen and numb. I hear buzzing, hissing, and extremely high-pitched noises. I am hot all the time and dripping wet with sweat. I am burning up from the inside out. My heart pounds and I feel shaky. I can't remember simple things. I am exhausted.

I am angry and I throw fits of rage. "I need help!" I scream in between sobs to my husband. I don't know what I am doing. My frustration is building. Please, I beg, help me. Please help me get out of the tub and get dressed. I can't do it by myself. I don't remember how. I am weak, tired, desperate, and drained.

How do I walk? My left side won't move with the rest of my body. I feel my leg, yet it's like dead weight and tingly right next to me. I can't move it without telling myself to lift it up. What's happening to me?

My short-term memory is failing. I can no longer concentrate. I did just put the conditioner in my hair, right?

I am "bedridden" without a bed. For three and a half months, in between trips to local doctors, I spend my days and my nights flat on my back, in the dark, on a futon mattress on the floor in our living room. I can't walk up the stairs to my bed. My body and brain won't allow it. I am too weak, my muscles are stiff, and I am extremely fatigued. Fear grips me. The life that I once knew is gone. And I know deep down in the core of my being that something is really wrong with me. I am trapped in a body that is no longer my own.

I can't go to work, can't read, can't write, and can't watch television. I cry every day after my husband leaves for work, and I remain here in the dark on this futon mattress on the floor. I contemplate suicide several times. I never truly believe that I want to die—although my daily pain is unbearable—and if God willed death upon me, I would welcome it.

My husband Josh, who is a teacher, comes home from work. He is worried about me. The next morning, he can't believe what he sees. This is not the woman he married.

He sees that my face has sagged. I cry out to him that my left side is numb, including my eye, tongue, and face, all of it from head to toe. It is 5:00 AM. He calls my doctor's answering service and leaves a message. In another fifty minutes, he will leave for work, an hour's commute by car, and I will be home alone, again. I am afraid. I don't want him to leave me.

He decides not to go to work, instead, he arranges for a substitute teacher to take over his classes, and brings me to a neurologist.

The neurologist's findings, a rare illness called CADASIL, prompt our Mayo Clinic visit. CADASIL stands for cerebral autosomal dominant arteriopathy with subcortical infarcts and leukoencephalopathy. It is a disease of young adults and presents with migraines with or without an aura, mood disturbances, focal neuralgic deficits, strokes, and dementia. It is a condition that leaves you facing migraines in your twenties, mini-strokes in your thirties, and then death by your forties. I want a second opinion. I *need* a second opinion. This *can't* be me, my life!

Josh packs the car and drives us to Mayo Clinic. We leave early on Saturday morning and arrive late on Sunday night. We arrive as walk-ins. The drive is long and painful, but we figure that I have nothing to lose.

It's Monday 7:30 AM, Minnesota time. We decide that we will wait as long as it takes to be seen, be it a week or a month. It doesn't matter, because I am not getting better in Michigan. I have had tons of tests done in the past seven weeks—MRI, sinus CT, two spinal taps, and a battery of blood and urine tests. I have tried several migraine medications; nothing works.

At Mayo Clinic, the only conflict that we have is my husband's work schedule. He arranges for a week off, something that is difficult to do when you have classes and students who depend on you. I think to myself, *If I don't get seen this week, I am in trouble.*

I am unable to read, write, or follow directions by myself. This mysterious illness forces me to be needy. I need my husband here with me. I—Ms. Independent World Traveler—can't even find my way around Mayo Clinic or read my testing instructions. He fills out my medical forms for me. I need help with everything these days: taking a shower, brushing my teeth, getting dressed, and blow-drying my hair.

As we wait in the waiting room, I silently pray to myself, "Please, God and the universe, just let me be seen. I need answers as to what is going on with my body. Please, call my name next."

"Ms. Chantal Hoey-Sanders?"

Did I hear that correctly? We've only been here for an hour and a half. It's not supposed to work like this. *Oh, God, I must really be sick! That tiny blue slip of paper that we filled out listed my top three symptoms,* I think. *I must really have something rare.*

*Thank you, MESSA health insurance, God, and the universe,* I silently say to myself as my name is announced through a microphone.

I am among two hundred or so other people in this room. We all sit here, in pain and in silence. The room reminds me more of a fancy bank than a hospital, with mahogany furniture from the late 1980s and shiny gray marble-tiled floors. The other patients all stare at me. I am the youngest in the room. I am the only one wearing sunglasses. I proceed to the counter.

Everyone at Mayo Clinic is very kind. They hand me a printout five pages long with times, locations, and test assignments on it. I can't read it. My husband reads it for me. He is my coordinator, my coach, my lifeline. I am thankful for him. I haven't always been thankful, I realize, and he hasn't always been like this with me either. In the beginning, the first month of my illness and inability to work, he—like countless others—thought that I was faking. He thought that this was some sort of a mental funk of mine to avoid going to work. I knew it wasn't.

This caused great tension in our fairly new marriage. We had been married only a year when I became ill. It wasn't until that morning—as I cried uncontrollably, when my husband saw that the left side of my face had slid and was sagging—that he finally believed me.

I have known all along that something was very wrong with me, with my whole being. I didn't need to look into the mirror and see my face to understand.

I go to Mayo Clinic twice. My initial trip is in October and Josh is by my side. The following month, I return to Mayo with the help of my caring mother-in-law for more extensive testing and MRIs with contrast dyes. Everyone at Mayo is very kind, and I am overwhelmed—in a good way—with their kindness. It is such an organized and well-run institution. It impresses me and I am hopeful.

But every day, this headache is getting worse. They say it is not CADASIL. Thank you, God and the universe! They conclude that it is classic migraine with prolonged aura, a condition that could lead into a stroke. I am to avoid caffeine, certain foods, to take one baby aspirin per day, and to follow the same rigid daily schedule.

I change my diet and I follow their guidance. "Make sure that you get at least eight hours of sleep per night," my doctor advises. *Yeah, right,* I say to myself, *I don't sleep.* My brain doesn't allow it and hasn't for the past twenty years. They give me the anti-depressant Trazadone for sleep and a laundry list of medications to try for the migraine. I diligently try each of these approaches over the next few months at home. None of them works.

My medical chart from Mayo Clinic reads as follows: severe migraine headaches with prolonged aura, polycystic ovaries, insulin resistance, and possible mood disorder. *"Depression" is what they mean by mood disorder,* I think, even though I have passed all my psychiatric evaluations with flying colors. This is not their final diagnosis; we are still waiting for more diagnostic tests to be taken and more samples to be returned before they draw any final conclusions.

## Understanding the Cause without Self-blame

It is now January. I am home alone in Michigan and have been here for the past five months. I have been sick since September and I am still in communication with the Mayo Clinic. As a follow-up they send bi-weekly urine and blood test "kits" to me. I take them to my local hospital's laboratory and have the samples drawn. My husband very graciously takes them to our local post office where they are returned to the Mayo Clinic for analysis. This continues for the next four months. I still don't have any concrete answers. I am housebound and unable to drive.

I take a medical leave from my job with the hopes of returning. I lose many of my friends. I don't blame them. No one knows how to help me, and rather than try, they avoid me. It is easier for them that way. My phone never rings.

I am forgotten. I am fragile. So many days, I struggle to catch my breath after standing up. It exhausts me. *Standing up exhausts me.* I need to rest, to lie down flat, just to catch my breath and to replenish my energy. What is wrong with me? I cry and I cry. I miss the life that has been snatched from me. I am stripped, exposed, and angry. I miss teaching and

I miss my students. I miss my independence and my mind. I feel reduced, dehumanized, pathetic. I feel like a failure.

This daily struggle between inner strength and outer dishevelment, pain, and fatigue is getting old. I try to rationally make sense of it and nothing comes to me. Nothing. I don't understand. Why me? How did I get here? Could it have been the accident on Labor Day at a local craft retailer that made me like this? Could this be because of the trauma that I received on the back of my head when one of the wooden displays fell and hit me? If that were the case, then why hasn't that shown up on any of my CTs or MRIs? I search my soul and press on with the nagging thought of *How did I get here?*

I get angry. My frustration fuels me, pushes me on, guides me aimlessly. I know that something is really wrong with my *whole being* and my body. For a short period of time, I disregard all of the medical journals, and I begin to take a huge look inward at myself. This inner spiritual journey is just about as scary as my medical one, yet I have a strong sense that they are connected and that I need to look inside of myself in order to truly become well. I need to figure out this disease. I am new to all of this, yet I am determined that I am going to figure this out if it's the last thing I ever do. My goal is simply to get to the bottom of this mysterious illness so I can find my cure.

Since I can't read, I call our local library and I order self-help books on CD and listen to them daily. Caroline Myss, John Kabbott-Zinn, and Louise Hay all become my steady companions. Their self-help tapes inspire me and help me to understand that all of my suffering may not be for naught.

For the first time in months, I feel that my struggle is going to help others. In fact, I sense through the center of my being that my struggle and my story are going to save others from the grief that I am experiencing right now. It's going to give them hope and help them. I'm not sure exactly how it will do this, but something deep down inside me knows it will.

I firmly believe that we go through good and bad experiences in life for a reason. The reason may not be known to us at the time, but it is there. I believe that we are here on Earth to live, to learn, to love, and to help each other. To me, there are no coincidences in life. When we know better, we do better. I also stand firm behind the power of positive affirmations and in creating your own hopeful and healthy destiny even when it looks grim. I did not ask to be sick. This is not the life that I had planned for myself, and although I have asked myself many times how I got here, I know that

I am not to blame. I am not the cause of my situation. I accept this now and say good-bye to my old life.

I have believed from the start of this illness, from the time when the doctors made their final diagnosis (no matter the diagnosis) that I *will* get well. I hold that power to get well. But first the doctors have to figure out what is going on with my body.

I try thirty different medications for my migraines, including some anti-seizure drugs and some anti-depressants; nothing works. I look normal on the outside, despite the fact that my body is screaming in pain. I always wear my sunglasses and a large-brimmed hat, even inside buildings. This illness is invisible, but I am not.

I am alone. My days drag on, as do my nights; I don't sleep. HSN, QVC, and my cats are now my only friends. I close my eyes in between commercials as the flashing lights from them are too blinding and painful for me to watch—small daggers piercing through my eyes. I no longer want morning to come. I even have the fleeting thoughts of praying for death, although this isn't truly what I want.

*I want to become well.*

## Saying Goodbye to the Old Life

Everything in my life is a struggle. In my world, the minutes feel like days, the days feel like months. I can't stand lying on this futon mattress on the floor any longer. Enough is enough. Something has to change. I search for the phone book. I force myself to read. I order myself a king-sized bed, mattress pad, and sheets. I pay for them by credit card, and I have them all delivered to our house. It's amazing how quickly beds can be delivered!

My husband arrives home to find a note posted on our downstairs den door: "Josh, I have a big surprise for you. I hope that you like it. *Je veux etre avec toi ce soir. Soyez heureux!*" (I want to be with you tonight, that is, in the same bed! Be happy.)

He is thrilled that he is home after his hour-long commute. He is relieved that I am still alive and that I haven't flooded the house. Yet, he is suspicious. He notices that I am dressed in street clothes, something he hasn't seen in months. In an instant, his face turns a ghostly sheet of white.

"You are up to something," he declares. "Oh my God, what have you done?" He rushes from the kitchen past the dining room into the living room. Then he sees my note taped to the den's door. He is *not* happy about the king-sized bed that now fills the whole space of our tiny den—but I am. As selfish as it is, this is my first step toward empowerment, wellness, and saying good-bye to my old life.

I am no longer able to teach. I extend my medical leave from my job with the now-distant hopes of returning. My assistant principal calls my house, but not to see how I am doing. Rather, he informs me about a rumor that is spreading around school that a student saw me at the movie theater last night with my family and that I did not appear sick. He said that I was not really sick and that I just didn't want to go to work!

Smart Alec. How rude and suspicious of him! After months of isolation my family had come into town for a visit and thought that it would be good for me to get out of the house and "do something fun." Little did they know the seriousness of my condition and the fact that I wouldn't be able to tolerate the flashing advertisements in the movie trailers. I wore my sunglasses and a large brimmed hat throughout the movie and decided that I won't be going back to any movies anytime soon. After that ordeal, I learned my lesson.

It is now May. Nine months have gone by—nine months of my precious life are gone. I take out our small town's phone book and begin my search. My sister Nicole, who lives in Florida, has mentioned several times to me now over the phone that I should try acupuncture treatments for my pain. She said that some of her friends have tried it for headaches and that it works. I should give it a try. I am leery about this hocus-pocus type of stuff.

"Now, what am I looking for?" I ask myself. "Acupuncture." I am drawn to one name. I have no idea why. It is a strange last name: Srutwa. I've never seen it before. I am clueless as to how to pronounce it. I completely struggle to read it.

I make an appointment with this MD acupuncturist. I very hesitantly tell this doctor my symptoms. I don't tell him everything all at once, for fear that he will think that I am crazy. I am *not* crazy. I am desperately searching for answers and hoping that someone will hear me and recognize what is going on inside my body.

The floodwaters are rising. I am waiting for the flood, hoping for a lifeboat, a lifejacket, something, anything. So many ships have passed me, and none has pulled me in. The water is ice cold and dark and I am drowning.

I am in his office. The lights are so bright. They're like small daggers piercing through my sunglasses and into my eyes. I am in pain. I shouldn't be here. He is taking my medical history. Does he hear me? Oh, God, the water is rising. I can't swim. *Please* help me!

My file is long. I reveal my stack of previous medical findings and X-rays. I am waiting for the flood. I hope that this doctor will be my lifeboat, the one who will tell me that I am not crazy, that dementia doesn't own me, that my body isn't falling apart, and that I am not dying. *I am not dying.*

My gown is a light cotton material, green in color, with a white trim around the edges and two ties on the back. The lights are off. A hint of daylight shines through the window blinds. Faint, soothing, rhythmic music is playing. An unfamiliar yet relaxing scent fills the air. The door is propped open. I sit and wait, sunglasses on, for the doctor to arrive.

He arrives. He is soft-spoken, kind, calm, professional, and serious. I begin to sweat. It trickles down my face, from my hairline, across my brow, and under my nose. I am embarrassed. I stammer to explain myself.

I am sinking deeper and deeper under the icy dark water. My body is struggling to come up for air. With moonlight as my only guide, I watch the bubbles drift effortlessly, one by one, to the top. I need to follow them, but I can't alone. Please, help me follow them!

## Getting Diagnosed

This doctor checks my muscles in two-inch increments. No other doctor has done this before. He very precisely and gently works his way from hand to shoulder, shoulder to hip, and hip to foot. I am perplexed, but I listen to him. I follow his orders. I make an appointment for next week.

Thursday arrives. I return. I am in his office. The lights are still too bright—small daggers that pierce through my sunglasses and into my eyes one by one. I am sweating and I don't understand why. I am soggy and chilled. The sweat covers me daily. I never get completely dry. I drip. I am embarrassed.

Again, I am sinking further and further under the icy dark water. My body is struggling to come up for air. The moonlight as my only guide, I watch the bubbles one by one drift effortlessly to the top. I need to follow them, but I can't alone. Please, help me follow them!

I Yahoo and I Google in between sobs and fits of rage, sunglasses on and middles of words missing. I force myself to read bits and pieces, links, and leftovers. Lyme disease? Lead poisoning? Fibromyalgia? Chronic fatigue syndrome? Multiple sclerosis? CADASIL? They all have similar symptoms.

I review my life, my medical history. All of these, I believe, are possible answers—except for the last two. Mayo Clinic ruled out multiple sclerosis and CADASIL. Thank God and the universe!

It is now June. Every day, this headache is getting worse. My ears are ringing; my eyes can't tolerate any light. The left side of my face and body are still frozen and numb. I hear buzzing, hissing, and extremely high-pitched noises. I am exhausted. My bladder is out of control. My fingers feel like they are the size of hot dogs. I can't open or extend my fingers. They are too stiff. What is happening to me? I have shooting pain. Stabbing and burning pain that travels throughout my body. I am dizzy and my perception is off. I frequently find myself walking into walls and furniture. My vision fades in and out and I have daily migraines with auras. These auras are visual disturbances that sometimes appear as flashing or zigzag lines in my visual field. Most of the time however, for me, they appear as temporary blind spots in my vision. Sometimes I lose my peripheral vision. They can last for twenty minutes or longer and usually, but not always, present with migraine headache pain. Auras terrify me and leave me feeling completely helpless. I want my old life back.

I don't want to do this anymore. I can't do this anymore. The doctors don't know what to do with me. They want to help me, but they don't completely believe me. I feel alone and hopeless. I just want out of this life.

Again, I contemplate suicide several times. I think about Jack Kevorkian, but he is now in jail. An aspirin overdose might work. But then if it doesn't completely work, my life will surely be no good to anyone. I could slit my wrists, but that would be too bloody and painful—and not fair to Josh. I know: I will walk out into the street and wait for an oncoming car to come and hit me. No; that's not fair to the driver of the car either. Obviously, I don't want to go this route.

I don't really want to die—I just want answers. I need to figure out what is wrong with me first, so I can find a treatment. I will get better. I will find my own cure if it is the only thing I do. I want my old life back. I will get better, no matter how long it takes me. I now live for Thursdays to arrive.

I return. I am in his office. The lights are so bright—small daggers that pierce through my sunglasses and into my eyes one by one. I am sweating and I don't understand why. I am soggy and chilled. The sweat covers me daily. I never get completely dry. I drip. I am embarrassed. I am on the examination table, with my sunglasses and green gown on.

## Finding Hope

I confide in this doctor that I can't remember simple things. I ask him if he thinks that dementia is beginning to own me. He tells me that this is something called fibro-fog. I am relieved. *Fibro-fog* doesn't sound like dementia to me. He explains that it is a combination of lack of sleep, the brain's inability to restore itself at night, and my diet. I might be hypoglycemic. I respond with, "Hypoglycemic? No, I have been tested for it many times and my tests are always negative." He informs me that the tests aren't accurate and that the only way I will really know for sure is by changing my diet. With beads of sweat forming on my forehead, I intensely listen.

I am hung up on one new term: fibro-fog. At this moment, it is the only thing that I hear in my head. It plays over and over again. My brain is stuck on repeat mode. I am not hearing another word this kind doctor is saying to me. My mind is racing, searching, scanning. I reflect on my Yahoo and my Google searches, and as a chill overcomes me, I realize—in an Oprah "aha" moment—I have fibromyalgia!

I am relieved. I am happy to have a name for this illness. Now I can find my treatment and my cure! This doctor proceeds with the acupuncture. I say nothing.

Before I leave, he hands me a book. It is white and green with white and blue lettering. I struggle to read it. *What Your Doctor May Not Tell You about Fibromyalgia,* by R. Paul St. Amand, MD and Claudia Craig Marek. I chuckle to myself at how appropriate the title is. I have been from neurologist to endocrinologist to psychiatrist to specialist after specialist—and none of them ever mentioned fibromyalgia to me.

The fresh spring flowers are starting to emerge. Lightness fills the air. Birds are chirping and squirrels are frolicking. I have a diagnosis that might actually explain all of my strange symptoms. I am on my road to recovery. Things are looking up. I have a diagnosis and that means that I can finally find a cure. I am happy, yet I am sad and perplexed for I am still sick. Spring break has come and gone and I haven't returned to work yet, though my job used to be my whole life.

Every shred of my self-esteem revolved around my work as a high school Spanish teacher. I lived and breathed it. I loved it, felt it my life's calling. I went back to school and sought another degree to become a teacher at the age of twenty-seven. As I write this, I am now thirty-two years old. I'm too young, not ready to watch my dreams painfully slip away. However, I finally have an official diagnosis and that means hope and recovery! I intend to get better. I intend to become well.

# Part 2

## Reducing Fibromyalgia Symptoms with Diet

# Chapter 2: The Second Step: Empowering Self

"When scientific literature says something is impossible, you have to create possibilities that don't exist yet."

—Dr. Robert Langer, professor, researcher, inventor, author

## Controlling Symptoms with Food: The Hypoglycemic Diet

I open the book, *What Your Doctor May Not Tell You about Fibromyalgia* (by R. Paul St. Amand, MD and Claudia Craig Marek), and search its table of contents. I go to chapter one, which is entitled, "An Invitation to Join Us and Find Your Way Back to Health." I like the name of this chapter. It's uplifting and inspiring. By the time I get to the second paragraph, I am hooked. The tears of a deep inner knowingness start to flow as I proceed to read the following paragraph:

> It can start out subtly: a bit of a muscle spasm, along with some generalized aches and stiffness. Then there are periods when concentration is impossible, a day or two of overwhelming fatigue, and maybe a little dizziness, some cramps and diarrhea. Symptoms come and go at first, and it's easy to chalk them up to a mild case of the flu that never quite hits. You may blame stress or overexertion for these strange little complaints. Then, one day, you realize one part or another of your body always hurts. Your life has entered a vortex, a downward spiral into more pain, depression, and fatigue.

I need not struggle to read any further. Dr. St. Amand understands. He has stood exactly where I am standing now. He is a fibromyalgia survivor himself and an endocrinologist. He is an expert in the field of hormones and metabolic syndromes like diabetes. I can't imagine a better teacher. Now it's my job to learn how I can get well with food, not pills.

I decide to start by reading only the section on hypoglycemia and diet. I realize that I will be reading all of the chapters eventually and that getting well with the Guaifenesin Protocol is five pronged: the Guaifenesin, the hypoglycemic diet, the salicylates, the symptom journal, and the mapping. But for now, since I am still struggling to read and to comprehend, I will focus all of my attention on my most pressing issues: my diet and how it relates to my fibromyalgia fog (fibro-fog), my migraines, my irritable bowel syndrome (IBS), my insomnia, my anxiety, my fatigue, and my constant sweating.

I skip to chapter five, "Hypoglycemia, Fibroglycemia, and Carbohydrate Intolerance." My newly diagnosed fibro-fogged brain struggles to read. But I know that if I am going to get well, this is what I must do. This is how I am going to get my life back. This is my step two.

I am familiar with the term "hypoglycemia." When I was in high school, my doctor suspected that I was hypoglycemic (or had low blood sugar levels) so he ordered the five-hour glucose tolerance test. Vividly, I remember sitting in the doctor's office and having to chug a large bottle of sweet orange-flavored syrup. Next, the nurse came in and took my blood; she would continue to do this every hour or so for the next five hours. Within seconds of drinking that horrible liquid, my heart started to pound and I started to sweat. I felt panicky and I developed a throbbing migraine in my left eye that made me dizzy and nauseated and sensitive to the lights in the office. I couldn't keep my composure. Other patients were staring at me, wondering what was going on. I thought that I was going to die. But I didn't die. In fact, my results came back negative. Negative! How on Earth could my results have come back negative? Within that five-hour time frame, my symptoms after drinking glucose were very severe: shakiness, sudden anxiety, heart palpitations, faintness, dizziness, nausea, facial flushing, sweating, and migraine headache. I swore to myself then and there that I was never going to take that test again—ever. What I've learned since that day is that the five-hour glucose tolerance test is severely flawed in testing for hypoglycemia. In other words, it is not accurate. The best way to test if you are truly hypoglycemic is to monitor your own symptoms after not eating for a few hours. How do you feel? Are you fatigued? Do you have a headache? Do you crave protein? Are you craving something sweet for a quick pick-me-up? If you start to feel weak, shaky, dizzy, nauseated, anxious, or tired, or start to sweat, develop heart palpitations, or get a headache, you may be hypoglycemic.

So here I am, twenty years later. I have made a complete circle. I am now on step two of finding wellness. I need to figure out which foods trigger my hypoglycemia (low blood sugar) and which foods will stabilize it. In order to do this, I will have to further study chapter five, "Hypoglycemia, Fibroglycemia, and Carbohydrate Intolerance" (from the *Revised and Updated What Your Doctor May Not Tell You About Fibromyalgia*, by Marek and St. Amand, 2006).

## Summarizing Dr. St. Amand's Theory of Hypoglycemia

(Quoted and reproduced with permission from the authors; www.fibromyalgiatreatment.com)

> The word hypoglycemia simply means low blood sugar. It's often used to suggest a disease but it is actually only one symptom of a syndrome with many complaints. This complex would be better defined by the term carbohydrate intolerance. It is expressed by the body's inability to use certain carbohydrate loads effectively without adverse consequences.
>
> When consumed, sugar and complex carbohydrates evoke a rise in blood sugar that triggers insulin release from the pancreas. This hormone facilitates immediate carbohydrate utilization or storage in various parts of the body. The liver converts excesses to fatty acids that are packaged into triglycerides and transported into fat cells for storage. In hypoglycemics, insulin release is either excessive, or the cutoff is inadequate, or insufficiently terminated by counter regulatory hormones. A system-wide disturbance is created that results in one of the endocrine fatigue syndromes we call hypoglycemia.
>
> The standard for diagnosis has been the five-hour glucose tolerance test (GTT). This was designed to document the rise and gradual fall of blood sugar after carbohydrate consumption. A sugar solution is administered and blood

samples are drawn at various intervals. The GTT has not been very efficient in detecting the sudden fall of blood sugar levels that characterize hypoglycemia. Timing is crucial and with predetermined schedule for blood draws, the lowest level may be missed. Another problem was seen in a study done in 1994 by Genter and Ipp on a group of young, healthy people who had no symptoms of hypoglycemia.[1] Blood samples were drawn every ten minutes to measure the amount and time-release of various hormones that counteract insulin to prevent an excessive drop in blood sugar. One-half of the subjects developed acute symptoms of hypoglycemia near the peak adrenaline release coinciding with their lowest glucose levels. However, the symptoms occurred at glucose levels that are considered normal. Obviously each person has a personal alarm system, an individual blood sugar level at which the brain perceives danger and releases adrenaline (epinephrine). For these reasons, listening to a patient's symptoms has been more accurate in making the diagnosis than blood testing.

The symptoms of hypoglycemia (a term we continue to use) are many. First are the chronic symptoms that are experienced even when the blood sugar is normal. They consist of fatigue, irritability, nervousness, depression, insomnia, flushing, impaired memory and concentration. Anxieties are common as are frontal or bi-temporal headaches, dizziness, or faintness. There is often blurring of vision, nasal congestion, ringing in the ears, numbness and tingling of the hands, feet or face and sometimes leg or foot cramps. Excessive gas, abdominal cramps, loose stools or diarrhea are frequent.

The acute symptoms are frightening and occur at highly variable glucose levels, but usually three or four hours after eating. The release of adrenaline, more than sufficient for correcting the fallen blood or brain sugar, induces these distressing twenty-to-thirty minute events. They include hand or internal shaking accompanied by sweating, especially with hunger. Heart irregularities or pounding and severe anxiety completes the picture. The more intense bouts are labeled panic attacks. Feeling faint is common and actual syncope may occur. Nocturnal attacks are often preceded by nightmares and cause severe sleep disturbance resulting in daytime somnolence.

Only a perfect diet will control hypoglycemia. It is not the food one adds but what one removes that assures recovery. Patients must totally avoid sugar, corn syrup, honey, sucrose, glucose, dextrose or maltose. Heavy starches such as potatoes, rice and pasta are also forbidden. We allow one piece of fruit in a four hour period but no juice since they contain excess fructose. Certain carbohydrates such as sugar-free bread are allowed but intake is limited to one slice three times per day. All carbohydrates are not created equal as can be seen by our list. You must follow the diet as written with no substitutions: for example puffed rice is allowed but not rice. Caffeine is not allowed since it prolongs the action of insulin.

Improvement begins in about seven to ten days of beginning a perfect diet. Considerable relief is afforded within one month**. Symptoms totally clear within two months but only if the diet has been carefully followed.** During the first ten days of treatment, headaches from caffeine withdrawal and the fatigue induced by changing the body's basic sources of fuel are common and in some patients can be fairly intense.

Consider the entire dietary process as if one were building a checking account. First, deposits must be made to obtain sufficient funds. Only at this point should one begin writing checks but with the understanding that balances are lowered with each one written. Similarly, the hypoglycemia diet builds energy reserves to the highest amount attainable for a given individual. Only then can carbohydrate experimentation begin. Each "cheat" draws on the credit line. Since no physician or dietician can predict the final baseline diet, this hunt and peck system is necessary for each patient. The first warning of an excess may be spotted with the reoccurrence of any of the above hypoglycemia symptoms. A stricter diet may again be required to rebuild credit, or to meet demands for added

> energy at times of emotional or physical stress such as during the week premenstrually.
> Some hypoglycemics also suffer from fibromyalgia. Symptoms overlap greatly but not the acute ones listed above. Fibromyalgia is a generalized metabolic disturbance that includes contracted, working muscles, ligaments and tendons, which constantly burn fuel. This is the subject of another paper we have written. Predisposed individuals with fibromyalgia may attempt to create energy by yielding to their carbohydrate cravings. The resulting repetitive insulin bursts can tip them into hypoglycemia. Patients with both conditions are among our sickest.

Although it's hard for me to completely wrap my brain around his theory, it does make sense to me. I must be hypoglycemic. I've always known instinctively in the past that when I would get a migraine headache, my body would always crave protein. I would either eat a hunk of cheese or a hamburger from Wendy's, and my headache would resolve itself within minutes. Unfortunately, this is not so anymore.

Now that I have an idea of how my body relates and reacts to my food intake, my goal for the day is to make a shopping list comprised of only my newly allowed foods. I realize that Dr. St. Amand has created two diets that both control blood sugar. They are called the strict diet for hypoglycemia (HG, or hypoglycemic, Strict Diet) for weight reduction, and the liberal diet for hypoglycemia (HG Liberal Diet.) I will stick to the strict HG side of the diet. When Josh gets home from work, I will talk to him about what I have learned, get his reaction, and present him with my list and our new lifestyle change.

I am lucky. Josh has decided to do the diet with me for the first three months, on the agreement that he is allowed to have two carb-loaded meals per week. I am thrilled to have his support, and I agree to his terms. I will stick to the strict end of the diet for myself, and he can do the strict side plus his two meals per week as he wants. We will begin in one week when he gets out for summer vacation.

## Preparing the Pantry: The Hypoglycemic Way

This shift in the foods that we are now going to eat feels enormous and overwhelming at times. I decide the easiest way to figure out how to welcome it into our lives is to replace all of the starchy foods on our plates that we used to eat with an allowed vegetable. That means broccoli will be substituted for rice, cauliflower for bread and rolls, and zucchini squash for pasta. Lettuce will replace the bun on my sub sandwich and hamburger. I will order my favorite taco salad without the onions, taco shells, refried beans, and rice. I will eat only the toppings on pizza, not the crust or sauce, and add a side salad. Good-bye heavy carbohydrates—hello health!

Josh helps me clean out our cupboards. I figure that this is the best way to ensure my success. We donate the "forbidden" foods that we are no longer going to eat to a local food pantry.

Next, Josh takes the grocery list to the store and shops for us because I am too sick to accompany him. He shops only the perimeter of the store, where all of the whole foods are located. He is not to go down any of the aisles, with the exception of frozen fruits and veggies, because this is where most of the heavy, carbohydrate-laden foods are located. Absolutely nothing sweet is to touch his cart.

We stock up on the allowed frozen veggies, frozen chicken breasts, lettuce, salad greens, Egg Beaters, eggs, cheese, cantaloupe, strawberries, nuts, olive oil, and fresh meats and fish. I have my husband order some tools for us: *What Your Doctor May Not Tell You about Fibromyalgia Fatigue* because I have heard that it is full of simple and easy recipes; a large wok-type pan for the stove; two lettuce spinners; two metal veggie steamer pan inserts; Solgar low-carbohydrate vanilla whey protein powder; Hefty zippered freezer bags; snack-size plastic baggies; and some of the clear glass Pyrex storage containers that go from oven to fridge. I put a food processor, a George Foreman Grill with removable plates, and the Magic Bullet personal blender on my birthday and Christmas lists—and hope that Santa will be good to me. These are our staples. I am ready to begin.

I will be honest with you. I am not fond of diets, and that is putting it very politely. I have struggled with my weight my whole life and have been on diets since the fifth grade. My mom tried hard to spare me the pain and anguish of being an obese child in a thin-obsessed society. To complicate my weight matters, I also have asthma and wasn't able to get much exercise growing up. Then, during my teen years, I outgrew some of my allergies and played tennis in high school. Consequently, I ate a banana and I drank a small can of tomato juice for lunch in the fifth grade. By the sixth grade, I had progressed to lunch consisting of one cup of yogurt with fruit on the bottom (360 calories, thank you).

My mom did the best she could. However, I won't go into details of the years that followed and my own self-struggles, self-hatred, and guilt with food, my weight, and anorexia. I only mention this now as the subject of hypoglycemia, diet, and fibromyalgia are so closely intertwined. Is hypoglycemia the reason why I have been plagued with weight gain, migraines, irritable bowel syndrome, insomnia, constant hunger, and sudden anxiety my entire life? Or could this have been the fibromyalgia all along? Maybe it was a mixture of the two conditions.

## Starting the New Lifestyle of Eating

I begin the strict diet for hypoglycemia because I need to lose weight. My first three days are hell. I am hungry *all* of the time. I can't stop thinking about what, where, and when I am going to eat next. I follow the book's guidance and eat when I am hungry; a little good fat like olive oil, avocado, canola oil, walnuts, or almonds, and a little low-fat protein like a scoop of low-carbohydrate whey protein powder, chicken breast, turkey, or fish. I am careful to eat only twelve nuts per day. To curb my hunger pangs and feel more satisfied throughout the day, I usually mix a scoop of the low-carb Solgar whey protein powder with eight ounces of water and a splash of olive oil. I am not accustomed to this type of diet. I am not used to eating so often without bread, pasta, potatoes, beans, milk, rice, or corn.

I am irritable and hungry all day long. I feel like I want to hit someone. By day four, I am frantically searching all of our cupboards for any remaining scraps of food and carbohydrates that we may have overlooked in our purging phase of the pantry in preparation for this new way of eating. Josh isn't home right now, and it is a good thing.

Like an addict, I need my sugar fix! In the fury of my frantic search for sweets, I realize one fact: I have not sweated at all! And although I am determined to find the food, I am not feeling anxious. Unbelievable! For the first time in twelve months, my anxiety is gone.

## Experiencing Positive Results

By day five, I don't have any cravings at all, and I am not irritable. I squelch my remaining hunger by upping my water intake. I mix a scoop of low-carbohydrate whey protein powder and a teaspoon of extra virgin olive oil with eight ounces of water. This helps me feel more satisfied. For the first time in my life, this new diet hasn't riddled me with guilt, food deprivation, or self-hatred.

I actually like the feeling of empowerment that I am creating. I realize that this is a lifestyle change. It's no longer about my body image. This new way of eating focuses on my health and well-being. It's not about what I am giving up; it is about what I am gaining.

By week two, my husband notices that I am no longer agitated. I don't feel like I need to hit someone anymore when it is time for me to eat. I am eating all day long, and the weight is dropping off. Every two hours, I eat a little good fat and a little good protein (like avocado, twelve nuts per day, or olive oil). I drink at least eight glasses of water each day to stay hydrated. I eat loads and loads of low-glycemic veggies. I buy them frozen and I steam cupfuls of them in my stainless steel wok-type pan. Once they are cooled, I transfer them into the glass storage containers. I am always thinking of easier ways to do things while cooking.

As a way to help conserve my energy, I always keep two metal veggie steamer-pan inserts, a large wok-type stainless steel frying pan, a medium-sized saucepan, and a medium-sized stock pot on my stove for boiling eggs or steaming veggies. This helps reduce my fatigue while cooking. I have also taken the time to organize my kitchen so like items are all stored together. For example: my Magic Bullet personal blender is kept on my counter, and its supplies are all stocked in the same cupboard above it, right next to the whey protein powder, and I keep the scooper for the powder in the can. This provides easy access for making my morning protein shake. In fact, I buy extra measuring utensils at the dollar store and keep them with the items that need to be measured. In my fridge, each shelf is devoted to certain foods. All frozen veggies are grouped together in the freezer on the top shelf, and frozen meats are stowed underneath. I also plan a two-hour block for cooking, either on Sunday night or Monday morning, so I start my week with plenty of food prepared in advance. I cut up celery, broccoli, and cauliflower and keep them stored in the glass containers. I buy a family pack of chicken and bake it all at once. This provides three meals for the week: garlic green bean chicken stir fry, chicken taco salad, and chicken nuggets. I take a package of lean ground turkey and divide it into twenty squares with a knife. Next, I place these squares on the broiler in my oven or on my George Foreman grill. In ten minutes, I will have mini-turkey burgers. They immediately go into my glass food storage containers. Organization like this helps to motivate me to stay on track with the diet. It's a must to always have quick hypoglycemic diet-friendly foods on hand to avoid cheating. *To avoid binging and going off plan, never let yourself get too hungry.*

Over the course of the next year, I watch my triglycerides fall from 458 to 222 to finally 140 by diet alone. I lose forty pounds. (Most of this weight I had gained on prednisone.) My husband loses eighteen pounds in the first three months, and his restless leg syndrome is gone! He has more energy and more stamina. I no longer urinate fifty times per day and sixteen times per night. My irritable bowel syndrome is better. My acid reflux has improved. I no longer endure day or night sweats. My heart doesn't pound or flutter anymore either. Although I am still very sick, I am improving. This new regime is working. I am making it work!

My friends and family look at my diet with rolled eyes and skepticism. They have never heard of a low-carbohydrate, low-fat diet. They have watched me repeatedly, throughout my lifetime, try fad diet after fad diet, become anorexic and exercise bulimic. They are worried, I am not. I am living the positive results!

They all fear that I am being too extreme with what I am no longer eating—the carbohydrates and refined sugars. They encourage me to eat comfort foods in the form of sweets. I refuse. I have my own doubts from time to time about my new diet until my blood tests return and they are normal without the use of cholesterol reducing medications. My night sweats are gone as long as I get up and eat a slice of cheese during the middle of the night. (The protein stabilizes my blood sugar throughout the night and doesn't create the adrenaline rush and night sweats.) For the past twenty years, three o'clock in the morning has been my waking hour every night. Now I know why—blood sugar and hormonal shifts. My migraines are less severe—still daily, but improved. Although sleep is still a problem and I never feel completely rested in the morning, this is still a great improvement for me. My restless leg syndrome is completely gone. I am able to put sentences together once again. I am able to read and to write again. There really is something to this diet for hypoglycemia. It works. I am on my way to great health! I can feel it. I am rebuilding myself, reprogramming myself, and reframing my thinking toward food. Who would have thought? It's not easy to eat this way, but it is confirmation enough for me to continue.

My secret weapon is not viewing this diet as a "diet." I have been on too many diets to know that diets don't work for me. The very word "diet" itself automatically conjures up images of past attempts of starving myself and body image failure in my world. Food is no longer my enemy or my long-lost friend. It is here to nourish my body and to make me strong and clear-headed. I am becoming healthier every day. The fibro-fog is *not* going to return, as long as I continue eating this way. And this is the key to it: I must continue to eat this way if I want to think clearly and be able to put my sentences together. I am slowly getting my mind back, and I am determined that it is going to stay with me. I want to be headache-free. Someday I will be completely headache-free. I will persevere. "I am woman, hear me roar!"

If anyone had ever told me that my migraines were triggered by sugar, I would have told them that they were *crazy,* because sweet foods always made me feel *happy,* not sick. I also never would have believed that even complex carbohydrates like whole-grain breads and pastas would have made me feel so sick.

Josh and I had made the healthy switch to whole-wheat pastas and Boca Burgers and were living a nearly vegetarian lifestyle for two years when I crashed with my fibromyalgia. Heart disease runs in his family, and we wanted to be proactive and try to ward it off. So you can imagine my shock when I learned that I was carbohydrate intolerant. I now know better, and I notice within five minutes of eating even a bite of a granola bar, a whole-wheat cracker, or bread, that my stomach starts to bloat, I immediately have gas, and my face and chest both flush. I have learned that food did cause and trigger my daily migraines, bodily pain, irritable bowel syndrome, anxiety, insomnia, and night sweats.

However, it wasn't until I followed Dr. St. Amand's diet for hypoglycemia for a week and I eliminated *all* refined sugar (simple carbohydrates found in white bread, processed foods, sugary beverages, and candy) and *all* complex carbohydrates (whole grain and whole-wheat breads, pastas, corn, and rice) that I began to feel improvement. Even the smallest bite of a food not allowed on the hypoglycemic diet would send me into a tailspin, make my face flush, make me sweat, my migraines scream, and my pain levels soar. Not only did my body feel dizzy, weak, and shaky after a diet cheat, this cheat would also impair my concentration and memory, activate my irritable bowel syndrome, and keep me up all night with night sweats and a pounding heart. The next day I would also experience—without fail—heartburn, irritable bowel syndrome in the form of diarrhea, a migraine headache, increased pain levels, and fibro-fog. I have learned that I am definitely carbohydrate intolerant. I simply can no longer eat any of these foods. Although the concept of being carbohydrate-intolerant is still hard for me to grasp, my body certainly responds positively to this way of eating. Who would have thought that food could affect a person like this?

Dr. Srutwa, my local MD acupuncturist, knew it. He agrees completely with Dr. St. Amand's theory of hypoglycemia and eliminating certain carbohydrates to obtain positive results. He equates this carbohydrate intolerance to the "fight-or-flight" mechanism in our bodies. He said that what we feel is an adrenaline rush after we eat a forbidden carbohydrate. This panicky feeling is that of our bodies trying to push our blood sugar back up after it falls. This happens when we eat something sweet or starchy and our blood sugar rises. Added to the story are the misfiring of the counter-regulatory hormones adrenaline, cortisol, growth hormone, and glycogen. The falling blood sugar frightens the brain and triggers the horrible symptoms of hypoglycemia: hunger tremors, pounding heart, panic attacks, faintness, fainting, intense hunger pains, and intense sugar cravings. Those of us with fibromyalgia have a double whammy. Dr. St. Amand explains this in his book:

> To make matters more complicated and confusing fibromyalgia and hypoglycemia have the following overlapping symptoms: ringing in ears, weakness, fatigue, irritability, moodiness, nervousness, depression, insomnia, impaired memory, impaired concentration, anxiety, frontal headache (migraines), dizziness, blurred vision, numbness (face or extremities), abdominal cramps, gas, bloating, diarrhea, sugar craving, swelling, weight gain, generalized muscle stiffness, nasal decongestion, and leg/foot cramps.

Again I got lucky. My local doctor also understood very well that the only way I would know if this diet would work for me was by actually adhering to it *perfectly for two months,* just as written by Dr. St. Amand. He told me that the blood tests for hypoglycemia are inaccurate most of the time because our bodies have the ability to restore and correct themselves quickly, making the low blood sugar levels non-existent by the time the blood is drawn. However, in certain individuals, these low blood sugar levels are traceable, but as he explains it, the test is inaccurate over 40 percent of the time.

I was stunned to learn that this blood test was still the only means that the medical community has to diagnose hypoglycemia, even to this day. Another shocker that my local doctor, Dr. Srutwa, shared with me was that medical students aren't even taught about hypoglycemia as a stand-alone condition in medical school. In fact, the majority of the medical community doesn't believe it exists, even in this modern day and age. It's criminal.

Forty percent of us with fibromyalgia are also hypoglycemic, and even more have the milder carbohydrate intolerance. Anyway, we have two overlapping conditions that most of the medical community still chooses to ignore: fibromyalgia and hypoglycemia. I won't go into detail about how detrimental these two facts are for us. Rather, I will focus on the fact that I am very thankful to have found the hypoglycemic diet and two doctors who believe that my condition is real.

I have concluded that my body needs this diet, and I have decided that I am going to commit to it. I am determined to treat my symptoms with food, not pills, especially since I was on thirteen prescription medications all at once this past year, and *none* of them helped alleviate *any* of my symptoms. But it was the best that those doctors knew how to do. I am still grateful for modern medicine.

Breakfast is going to be my most challenging meal. I will have to give up my oatmeal and banana. Bye-bye milk, cereal, graham crackers, and toast. I will also need to change my thoughts about morning foods and eat items that I normally would not have considered as choices. It won't be easy. But I did learn to eat rice and fish for breakfast my year abroad living in Korea. There I realized that it's the morning foods that you are raised with that determine your concept of what to eat first thing after you wake up. In Korea, cereal and milk weren't an option, at least not with my host family. Sandwiches were foreign, too. So I know that I can do this! I can completely change my eating habits. I can change the way that I view sweet treats and food. They are no longer "treats" but rather things that feed my migraines, anxiety, brain fog, pain, and fatigue. If I want to remain symptom-free, I have to adhere to this new lifestyle of eating. My dad is a type-II diabetic, but he rarely watches his diet or tests his sugar. He tells me that a little sugar won't hurt me, yet he can't figure out why he has developed neuropathy in his feet! He thinks that amputation will never happen to him because he takes his medications for diabetes daily—all five of them! He doesn't believe that he can actually treat and possibly control his diabetes with food instead of pills.

This isn't going to be easy, but I am worth it. I know that I can do this. My thoughts about food are my power. I am in control. I am in charge. No tweaking or substituting. The more tired I may become directly after starting the diet, the more it means that I need it. Whether I actually am hypoglycemic or not is not the real issue here. The real issue lies in empowering myself through this new healthy lifestyle of eating and using it to get my life back. I won't let myself think that I am being deprived. I am not going there. The pity party down Sugar Street won't seduce me. This is not about what I am giving up (food wise), it is about what I am gaining (getting my life back). I will remember this and recite this affirmation whenever I start to falter. I will remind myself that I deserve perfect health. "You deserve perfection, Chantal." I will become my own cheerleader and wave my own pom-poms.

I will pay careful attention not to beat myself up if I eat something off plan. I know that I am human and that it will happen from time to time. Rather, I will learn from it and move forward. I won't let my slip-up hinder me from obtaining my goal: perfect health! I understand that this is a gradual process and that eating healthily will require more energy from me to cook and to prepare meals, and that is why I am starting out with mostly frozen items. I know that I am able to open a bag and throw hypoglycemic-friendly frozen foods into a pan, a microwave, or a steamer-pan insert. That much I can do!

My goal for each and every day is to prepare healthy meals for myself and my family—even if this is the only task that I am able to complete for that day. This is the most import step in reducing and controlling my hypoglycemic symptoms for my return to perfect health. These foods are my new medicine. They are going to be the fuel that I will need to reclaim my life. This is the investment that I must make right now in myself. I am not a cook, so this is going to be an adventure, the challenge of all challenges. All of my meals are going to be prepared from scratch. No boxed or pre-made anything. Yes, I can do this. Welcome to the kitchen of the world-famous chef Chantal, who has spent all day graciously preparing the most scrumptiously healthy meals for you!

My next step is to fill my cupboards with cooking utensils and baking items that help me preserve my energy and support me daily. Simplicity is the key. Objects like a salad spinner, clear Pyrex glass containers that go from oven to table to fridge, and a large stainless-steel frying pan with metal vegetable steamer-pan inserts will soon become my new best friends.

I will focus on preparing extra food for use as leftovers for breakfast or lunch the next day. By doing this, I am putting my health first. We will hold a family meeting to discuss nutrition and everyone's new role in helping me to get well. I will set aside my feelings of shame, guilt, and embarrassment. I will ask for assistance when I need it from family members or friends. Maybe they can shop for me.

Little by little, I will create a system and a plan. I will think ahead and devote two hours each Sunday night or Monday morning to cooking meat—a family pack of chicken to be used later in the week and mini turkey burgers and turkey meat loaf. I will boil a dozen eggs and make one crustless quiche and have them readily available. My goal here is to get well. I know that by fueling myself with the right foods—lean protein and low-glycemic fruits and vegetables, I will be able to get both my mind and body back.

No matter what, I will not give in to any of my own excuses of why I can't convert to this healthy way of eating. Monday will be fish night, Tuesday will be taco salad and homemade salsa, Wednesday will be turkey-stuffed peppers, Thursday will be chicken garlic green bean stir fry night, etc., and I will repeat these meals every week for the first month. I will not listen to my mind chatter that will tell me things like I am bored with this food or I don't feel like eating that meal. I will make food plans in advance, no matter how fatigued I am. I know that restoring my health revolves around getting my blood sugar stabilized. Maybe my husband Josh and stepson Nik can help me.

By following the diet exactly as written, I will no longer have spikes in blood sugar and the insulin release that creates our multitude of debilitating symptoms. All symptoms of blood sugar fluctuations will disappear. It sounds too good to be true, doesn't it?

But it is true! I quickly replace caffeinated beverages with Solgar low-carbohydrate whey protein powder. I make it routine to never leave the house for an appointment without first drinking a scoop of it mixed with eight ounces of water. I pack allowed nuts, slices of cheese, and mini-turkey burgers to bring with me on my outings. I have breakfast options prepared in advance because I always make sure that there are leftovers stored in my fridge in clear glass Pyrex rectangular containers or the like (so I can easily stack and identify food contents) from the night before. The more prepared in advance I am, the more successful I will be. The longer that I eat this way, the more energy I will have. (For more information on this subject, please refer to the *Updated and Revised What Your Doctor May Not Tell You About Fibromyalgia Fatigue.*) Eventually I may even be able to reverse my hypoglycemia and not become a type-II diabetic. Wouldn't that be wonderful?

The following is a list of the items from this chapter that I used to get started with the Strict Diet for hypoglycemia. Please keep in mind that both diets control blood sugar, although the Strict Diet is for weight loss only. The Liberal Diet is for weight maintenance. Enjoy and Be Well!

## Non-Food Items to Get You Started with the Strict HG Diet

- *What Your Doctor May Not Tell You about Fibromyalgia Fatigue,* by Claudia Craig Marek and R. Paul St. Amand MD
- A large frying pan or wok-type pan and lid (I always keep/stow my three pans on the stove top in order to preserve my own energy.)
- A large stock pot and lid for boiling eggs and steaming veggies like cauliflower and broccoli.
- A medium-sized sauce pan and lid.
- Two lettuce spinners. These are great for cleaning lettuce and other veggies. I also use them for both serving and storage.
- Four metal veggie steamer-pan inserts.
- Hefty zippered freezer bags.
- Snack-size plastic baggies.
- Clear glass rectangular (they stack well in the fridge) Pyrex food storage containers with lids that go from oven to fridge.
- A food processor for chopping veggies, making sugar-free salsas, and preparing whipped cauliflower.
- George Foreman Grill with the removable dishwasher-safe plates.
- Magic Bullet personal blender.

## Food Items

- Solgar (or similar) low-carbohydrate vanilla whey protein powder. Often I put it in my water bottle with eight ounces of water and one teaspoon of extra virgin olive oil and bring it with me and sip on it for the day.
- Frozen zucchini squash, broccoli, green beans, cauliflower, brussels sprouts, spinach, asparagus, and mixed peppers.
- Frozen cauliflower—See Whipped Cauliflower below.
- Frozen chicken breasts—I bake eight breasts at one time at 300° for 40 minutes in my large glass Pyrex baking pan and

once they are cooled I store them in the fridge. During the week I use this meat for salads, taco salads, and stir-fries.

- Frozen fish—salmon, tilapia, orange roughy, and cod.
- Lettuce and salad greens.
- Eggs—At the beginning of the week, I boil up a dozen and either keep them whole and eat only the egg whites or make egg salad with 2 egg yolks, 10 egg whites, chopped celery and sugar-free mustard and mayo.
- Egg Beaters — See Easy Crustless Quiche below.
- Cheese in brick form.
- Cheese, pre-shredded—great for salads and on top of the quiche.
- Cooking spray—olive oil.
- Cantaloupe—In a blender, mix ¼ cantaloupe wedge with 6 ice cubes and 1 scoop vanilla protein powder. Blend on high until frothy. Serve.
- Strawberries—In the Magic Bullet, combine 6 frozen strawberries, 1 scoop vanilla whey protein powder, and 8 ounces of water. Blend for 10 seconds. Serve. Alternate strawberries with cantaloupe and 6 ice cubes.
- Nuts, almonds, and walnuts—12 per day for weight loss—Roast your own in the oven. Place nuts on cookie sheet. Bake at 350° for 10 minutes. Rotate nuts every 3 minutes.
- Olive oil—This is the only dressing I use, sometimes mixed with apple cider vinegar. Newman's Own Organic Olive Oil is excellent!
- Fresh or frozen meats without added sugar—Always read food labels and ingredients. Manufacturers hide sugar in everything these days. Beware of ingredients that end in *-ose* (dextrose, sucrose, maltose, glucose, fructose, high-fructose corn syrup), honey, and cane juice.
- Jennie-O lean ground turkey—See Mini Turkey Burgers below.

## Quick and Easy No Fuss Recipes

- **Turkey Meat Loaf**—In a large bowl, combine two packages of Jennie-O lean ground turkey with four stalks of chopped celery and one bunch of green onions. Use food processor to chop celery and green onions before combining. Sprinkle on garlic and pepper to taste. Mix in bowl (I use my hands.) Spray oven-safe baking dish with Pam olive oil. Form ingredients into a loaf. Bake at 350° for 40 minutes. Pierce with a fork for doneness.

- **Turkey Stuffed Peppers**—Lightly oil frying pan with Pam olive oil cooking spray. Brown meat in frying pan until completely cooked. Add garlic powder and chili powder to taste. Combine one package frozen peppers to meat. Sprinkle olive oil over frozen peppers and toss. Add garlic powder and chili powder to taste. Let simmer until frozen peppers are cooked. Next, wash and core six peppers—2 yellow, 2 red, 2 orange. Cut each pepper in half lengthwise. Microwave peppers on high for 3 minutes or until cooked. Preheat oven to 350°. Finally, place one inch of water in the bottom of an oven-safe Pyrex baking dish. Set open-faced peppers in the dish. Stuff with turkey and pepper mixture. Add half slice of cheese if desired or sprinkle on parmesan cheese. Bake 10-20 minutes. Check to ensure cheese has melted and meal is hot and ready to serve. Enjoy!
- **Garlic Green Bean Chicken Stir Fry**—Coat large wok-style stainless steel pan with olive oil. Peel ten garlic cloves. (To save energy, time, and my fibromyalgic fingers, I buy these in bulk already peeled.) Add two stalks chopped green onions. Lightly brown in pan. Add pre-baked, pre-cut chicken (about 4 breasts). Chicken should be pre-cut into bite-sized pieces. (I usually cut my chicken right after I bake the family pack, and then I divide it into 4 breasts and store individually.) Cook chicken until heated. Add 4 cups frozen green beans. (I buy my organic beans in a large bulk bag.) Toss with olive oil and garlic powder. Cover and simmer until ready to serve. Enjoy!
- **Chicken Nuggets**—Lightly coat Pyrex baking dish with actual olive oil—not Pam spray! Place pre-cut, pre-baked chicken (about 4 breasts) in dish. With a fork lift chicken pieces and spread around to cover with olive oil. Sprinkle with oregano. Preheat oven to 350°. Bake for 40 minutes. Flip chicken pieces after 20 minutes and sprinkle on parmesan cheese. Enjoy!

- **Chicken Taco Salad—**Coat large wok-style stainless steel pan with extra virgin olive oil. Add pre-baked, pre-cut chicken. Sprinkle with chili powder to taste. Simmer on low until chicken is heated (around 20 to 30 minutes). Stir occasionally. Add more spices to taste. To prepare the salad: cut up lettuce, tomatoes, and avocados. Top with shredded cheese. If you have non-HG family members or you are on the liberal side of the HG diet, then you can also top salads with corn tortilla chips. Enjoy!
- **Whipped Cauliflower**— Steam one bag frozen cauliflower. Cool and add to food processor. Add four tablespoons Newman's Own Organic Extra Virgin Olive Oil. Blend together. Taste. Add more olive oil if desired. May also combine one fourth cup reduced fat shredded cheddar cheese or one fourth cup heavy whipping cream. Enjoy!
- **Easy Crustless Quiche**—Spray a 9x13-inch baking dish with Pam olive oil. Next pour one 32-ounce carton of Egg Beaters or 12 eggs into pan. Microwave one box of frozen spinach and one bag of frozen broccoli (or acceptable veggies of your choice) on high for 6 minutes. Drain excess water. Combine veggies and one-half bag shredded cheese and place into baking dish. Swirl with fork. Evenly mix eggs and veggies with cheese. Bake at 350° for 30 minutes. (For extra variety, you may add chicken, ham, walnuts, almonds, or anything you'd like that's on the diet. I usually make this every other week and eat it for breakfast or lunch.) Enjoy!
- **Mini-Turkey Burgers—**Open package. With a knife, divide turkey into 20 small squares. Cut 5 squares the long way and 4 squares the short way. Remove from package and place squares on the George Foreman Grill and cook for 10-12 minutes at 300°. Store in a glass Pyrex container. (These mini burgers are great for on-the-go snacks.) Enjoy!

## Diets for Hypoglycemia

by R. Paul St. Amand, M.D.

(Reproduced with permission from the authors; www.fibromyalgiatreatment.com)

Both these diets work to correct hypoglycemic (blood sugar) symptoms. Choose the strict diet to lose weight or the liberal diet to maintain weight.

You must do the appropriate diet AS WRITTEN for two months, without cheating. At that point, if you are on the liberal diet you can start to experiment with forbidden foods to see what you can tolerate.

Each hypoglycemic's tolerance for listed foods will vary. Judge your tolerance level by how you feel and adjust your intake of foods accordingly.

### The Strict Diet

Choose any foods from the following list

| MEAT and FISH |
|---|
| All meats except cold cuts that contain sugars or dextrose; All fowl and game; All fish and shellfish. |
| DAIRY PRODUCTS |
| Eggs; Any natural cheese (bleu, Roquefort, cheddar, cream, gouda, swiss, etc;) Cream (heavy and sour;) Cottage and Ricotta (1/2 cup limit per day;) Butter; Margarine. |
| FRUITS |
| Fresh coconut; Avocado (limit 1/2 per day;) Cantaloupe (limit 1/4 per day;) Strawberries (limit 6-8 per day;) Lime or Lemon juice for flavoring (limit 2 tsp. per day.) |

### VEGETABLES

Asparagus; Bean Sprouts; Broccoli; Brussels sprouts; Cabbage (limit 1 cup per day); Cauliflower; Celery Root (celeriac;) Celery; Chard; Chicory; Chinese cabbage (limit 2 cups per day;) Chives; Cucumber; Daikon (long, white radish;) Eggplant; Endive; Escarole; Fennel Bulb; Greens (Mustard, Beet, Collard etc;) Jicama; Kale; Leeks; Lettuce (any type;) Mushrooms; Okra; Olives; Parsley; Peppers (green, red, yellow, etc;) Pickles (dill, sour, limit one per day;) Pimiento; Radicchio; Radish; Rhubarb; Sauerkraut; Scallions (green onions;) Spinach; Squash (yellow or summer only;) String beans (green or yellow;) Snow peas; Soy Beans, Tomatoes (not sauce or paste); Water Chestnuts; Watercress; Zucchini.

### NUTS (limit 12 per day)

Almond; Brazil; Butternut; Filbert; Hazel; Hickory; Macadamia; Pecan; Pistachio; Sunflower seeds (small handful); Walnut.

### DESSERTS

Sugar-free Jell-O; Custard (made with cream and artificial sweetener.)

### DRINKS

Club soda; Decaffeinated coffee; Decaffeinated tea; Caffeine-free diet sodas.

### CONDIMENTS and SPICES

All herbs and spices including seeds (fresh or dried); All imitation flavorings; Horseradish; Sugar-free sauces such as Hollandaise, Mayonnaise, Mustard, Ketchup; Sugar-free salad dressings; Oil and Vinegar (all types;) Worcestershire sauce.

### MISCELLANEOUS

All fats; Caviar; Tofu.

FOODS TO STRICTLY AVOID

Alcohol (most hypoglycemics can tolerate one drink after two months on the diet - use discretion as individual tolerance levels vary;) Baked beans; Refried beans; Black-eyed peas (cow peas); Bananas; Lima beans; Potatoes; Corn; Dried fruits and Fruit juices; Barley; Rice; Pasta (all types;) Flour and Corn Tortillas; Tamales; Sweets of any kind; Products which contain Dextrose, Glucose, Hexitol, Lactose, Maltose, Sucrose, Honey, Fructose, Corn Syrup, Food Starch, Agave Nectar, Caffeine.

## The Liberal Diet

You may add the following foods to the strict diet:

FRUIT

(limit: one piece of fruit every four hours. No fruit juices.)
Apples; Apricots; Blackberries (1/2 cup limit;) Blueberries (1/2 cup limit;) Boysenberries; Casaba melon (1 wedge limit;) Grapefruit; Honeydew melon (1 wedge limit;) Lemons; Limes; Nectarines; Oranges; Papaya; Peaches; Pears; Plums; Raspberries; Strawberries; Tangerines; Tomato juice; Tomato sauce or paste; V8 Juice.

VEGETABLES-remove limit from strict side

Artichokes; Beets; Carrots; Onions; Peas; Pumpkin; Winter squash; Hubbard squash; Turnips; Rutabagas, Spaghetti squash.

NUTS—no limit

Cashews; Peanuts; Soy Nuts.

DAIRY PRODUCTS

Whole, Non-fat, Low-fat milk and buttermilk, unsweetened yogurt.

DESSERTS

Sugarless diet puddings (1/2 cup a day limit)

| BREADS |
| --- |
| Three slices a day of sugar-free white, whole wheat, sourdough or light rye. No more than two slices at one time. |
| MISCELLANEOUS |
| Corn tortillas (2 only per day;) Carob powder; Flour (gluten or soy only;) Gravy made with gluten or soy flour only;) Popped popcorn (one cup only;) Sugar-free cereals (puffed rice, shredded wheat, oatmeal etc;) Wheat germ. |

If cholesterol is a problem, avoid cold cuts (except turkey,) cheese, cream, solid margarine, hollandaise sauce, and macadamia nuts. Use egg whites or Egg Beaters instead of whole eggs. Use liquid margarine only. Nuts should be dry-roasted only. Trim all visible fat from meats and remove skin from poultry. Use canola or olive oil.

*This diet is not meant to be used as to make a medical diagnosis. Please consult your own physician before making any changes to your current diet, medications or treatment. Prior to commencing any diet, R. Paul St. Amand MD recommends a basic work-up that includes a thyroid test, blood count, blood-glucose screening, and testing for any conditions that may mimic blood sugar abnormalities.*

# Part 3

## Reclaiming Self

# Chapter 3:
# The Third Step: Adjusting to the New Life

"And the day came when the risk it took to remain tight in a bud was more painful than the risk it took to blossom."

—Anais Nin

I recognize you. In this moment, you are feeling as if you have been reduced to nothingness, although you haven't. Most likely, you have gone from doctor to doctor, spent thousands of dollars, gotten your diagnosis, and tried almost every possible promised imaginable fibromyalgia /chronic fatigue syndrome cure. Nothing has worked, and your relationships have suffered. With looming feelings of despair, you continue to long for that old life.

You are currently at the worst stage of your illness, and the prospect of wellness has escaped you. But I can tell you it is going to get better. You are going to succeed. You don't realize it now, but you will surmount this illness as a much better and stronger person. You must have blind faith, patience, and determination. You now have hope. I am living proof of it. You may have fibromyalgia/chronic fatigue syndrome, but it doesn't have you!

The mere fact that you are reading this book right now proves that you have already begun to take charge of your health and that you are not allowing yourself to play the victim. You are stronger than you think. You hold the power to get well. So believe in yourself and take that giant leap. Join me in the reversal process. Let's journey together.

## Remembering the Old Life

My life as a high school Spanish teacher was vibrant and colorful. I enjoyed teaching, and although I had struggled with daily migraines for the past twelve years, I never imagined that one day they would flatten me and rip me away from my classroom. I will never forget that day—a warm and sunny Tuesday, the day after Labor Day in 2002.

I was in the middle of teaching my fifth-hour Spanish class. We were playing a verb game and laughing and having a great time. Life was good until one of the fluorescent ceiling lights began to flicker. At first, I thought nothing of it, and we continued with our fun. Within seconds, however, I was struggling. My brain was playing tricks on me by presenting me with a shimmery aura and partial vision loss that forced me to immediately teach from a chair.

I explained to my students that I was having a migraine and that I hoped it would resolve itself. I excused myself and proceeded to my desk, where I quickly took an over-the-counter headache medication. With all thirty-three sets of eyes on me, the painful throbbing began. It quickly pulsed its way up the back of my neck and clawed itself deep inside my temples, where it settled itself like a dagger behind my left eyeball. Suddenly I began to lose my speech and then more of my vision. My left side, including my tongue and face, went numb. My words became jumbled. I could only see partial images, not the whole. This made me feel off-balance. I was worried. Was I having a stroke? Or was this my usual migraine with aura?

I knew I was in trouble as soon as I felt my tongue go numb. We only had a few minutes left until class would be dismissed, and I tried to hide my fear and pain from my students. When the lunch bell finally rang, I managed to hobble into the classroom next door and alert another teacher that I needed help. I was having difficulty walking and seeing. Before I knew it, I was being wheeled out of the school and into the emergency room of our local hospital. Although I didn't realize it then, it was in that instant that my teaching days were finished.

The day before this episode at school, I had gone to a large arts-and-crafts retailer to pick up some teaching supplies. While I was there, one of their displays had fallen and struck me on the back of the head. Stunned and embarrassed, I did not file an incident report.

Although I can trace my fibromyalgia symptoms all the way back to infancy, and then later to a horseback-riding fall at age sixteen (when I noticeably received my first fibromyalgia lump in my right buttock), my final fibromyalgia/chronic fatigue crash arrived sixteen years later.

It's amazing how each of us with fibromyalgia can go back to that very moment when our lives changed forever. It could have perhaps been a physical trauma like mine, a virus, the birth of a child, or an emotional hardship. They all quickly propel you out into that vast sea and then leave you shipwrecked while the sharks circle.

Because teaching had been my life, I felt like a complete failure when I could no longer do it. I felt ashamed and worthless. I immensely enjoyed being in the classroom preparing and creating, and sharing my knowledge with my students. I spent many long hours counseling and consoling, and I prided myself on helping them learn and grow as individuals. I was always grateful that my students felt comfortable enough with me to visit me during my lunch period and after school. Often my classroom was filled with those curious individuals who didn't actually have me as a teacher. I was truly going to miss them and miss teaching.

However, I had to face the hard facts: I was no longer that person—the teacher—they once knew. Fibromyalgia, with all of its afflictions, widespread chronic pain and fatigue, daily migraines, irritable bowel syndrome, acid reflux, interstitial cystitis, insomnia, anxiety, vulvodynia, hypoglycemia, and fibro-fog had quickly made sure of that for me.

Languages were *my thing*. I loved them, and I loved grammar. I memorized easily. I spoke French, Spanish, English, and Korean, so you can only imagine my horror when the fibro-fog took over my brain and I couldn't put a coherent sentence together in any of them.

With the onset of my fibromyalgia, my speech became jumbled. "Bundle up" became "buckle up." "Recreation" became "recognition." I would think that I was saying one word, yet another word would actually come out of my mouth. I was afraid. My neurologists feared that I might have had a mini-stroke and that further testing may reveal more. When all of my tests came back inconclusive, my doctors were perplexed. None of them suspected fibromyalgia.

While they couldn't completely rule out a mini-stroke, I now know that my memory and concentration problems (fibro-fog) were the result of a combination of lack of sleep, improper diet, and the chronic daily migraine. The headache pain that I felt alone was relentless and extended from inside my eyes, jaw, face, neck, and down my left side into my arm and leg.

## Accepting Disability, not Defeat

Physically, I knew that I was in trouble. I looked normal, but my body was screaming in pain. Emotionally, I was suffering terribly. Mentally, I was certain that I couldn't go back to work. I feared for myself, and my ego couldn't share with the rest of the world how plagued with failure and frustrated I felt. I could no longer remember simple things. Chapter 1 is a good example of what my world had become.

My fibro-fog was thick. My short-term memory and my ability to concentrate were literally gone. In fact, I was so fibro-fogged that I could no longer recognize my own street when my husband drove me down it. It may sound unbelievable, but it's true. This happened to me several times, and Josh always thought that I was joking. I wasn't. I was terrified. I knew that I could no longer teach or return to work with my memory like this. I had to face the facts.

Applying for social security disability income was another emotional issue I needed to tackle. Owning up to this fact meant that I indeed was no longer the person I used to be. The idea of being only thirty-two years old and on disability was humiliating. The very thought of applying for disability overwhelmed and insulted me. I am someone who doesn't like asking for help or feeling like a burden.

Mustering up enough courage to ask the doctors I was seeing if they would support my disability was one of my biggest emotional hurdles, but it was absolutely my next step toward recovery. I did not want to do this.

My already shy nature made it even harder for me. Then the voice of self-pity started to creep in. "This is not how my life was supposed to be. This is not the life that I planned. I want my old life back! I want to teach. I want to feel like I am making a difference. I do not want to be soaking off of the system. I don't want to be a failure. Not being able to do my job embarrasses and humiliates me."

Once again, the emotional issues were surfacing, and not being able to teach was huge. I was not ready to let go of my job. My life revolved around being a high school Spanish teacher. In reality, somewhere along the way, I had let my job define me, and saying good-bye to it was like pulling teeth from a wild tiger. What would I do with myself if I couldn't work? Who would I be if I wasn't a teacher?

## Believing in Self: Emotional Issues

I take a deep breath and a huge look inward. I let my anger and my despair fill me for a few seconds. I grieve. I know what needs to be done. With great hesitation, I ask my husband to help me. I need to apply for social security disability income. Although I am on the right track with reversing my fibromyalgia and I am becoming healthier every day, my reality is that I need to figure out how to pay the bills while I am getting well. After all, I don't know how long it will take to reverse my fibromyalgia.

Josh contacts my employer and requests that long-term disability papers be sent to our house. I know that I can't return to work yet. I accept it. I move forward. This is my now. When the forms arrive, I dictate the information to him, and he fills them out for me. I find this process overwhelming and need help. Although it has been a hard lesson in my fibromyalgia journey, I am realizing is that it is okay to ask for help—and to accept it. Josh makes another phone call and contacts the social security disability office and requests the forms for me. He sets up a time for a telephone interview. (This can now all be done online.)

At first, having my husband do these things for me humiliates me. I wish that I could do this for myself. Although I am very thankful for him and I love him dearly, the idea of not teaching leaves me feeling completely empty and abandoned. I feel lost. More soul searching and tears of frustration are needed. Does being on social security disability mean I am a failure?

My answers come slowly and with much resistance. After great debate, while talking to my husband and speaking with a family friend who is on disability, I finally reach the conclusion that applying for social security disability benefits doesn't mean that I am a failure. I was never my job, although I did get most of my self-worth from it. I am simply someone who has hit a bump in the road and needs assistance right now. I don't know what my future holds. All I have is this very moment, and right now, I need help. I am someone who has worked hard over the years. I have contributed successfully to society. I do deserve social security disability income, and I can prove my case. I will set my fears aside.

What I have learned—especially now, over the past eight years—is that I had to take baby steps back to wellness and that I needed to use any and all tools at my command. For me, this meant first cutting myself some slack, letting myself grieve my losses, and working through my anger and frustration. I had to come to terms with the fact that I was not my job.

Ouch! And that someone else could fill my job. Double ouch! And that I was not this illness. I suddenly had a huge space inside of me to fill.

I chose to fill it by focusing on the fact that while I can be *changed* by what happens to me, I can also refuse to be *reduced* by it. My paycheck did not define me, and being on social security disability income was not the end of my career. Rather, applying for SSDI is what I needed to do as a stepping stone to get well.

## Becoming the Change: Affirmations

Yes, home alone in pain, desperate and drained, I found ways to empower myself. I began by ordering free self-help books on tape from my local library, and I learned about the healing affects of positive affirmations. I taught myself how to do guided imagery and meditation. I listened to these books on tape and practiced daily. Slowly, I created the change in myself that I wished to see.

Louise L. Hay; Jon Kabat-Zinn, PhD; Judith Orloff, MD; Emmett Miller, MD; and Caroline Myss all became my steady companions. Whenever I felt myself becoming anxious, discouraged, trapped, and feeling worthless about my life and my health (and it did creep in more than I liked), I would reflect on their teachings and repeat over and over to myself the following quotes and positive affirmations:

**"I can be changed by what happens to me, but I refuse to be reduced by it." —Maya Angelou** (My all-time favorite. This quote got me through the days when I was first ill and I cried every day in the mornings after my husband left for work.)

**"I return to the basics of life: forgiveness, courage, gratitude, love, and humor." —Louise L. Hay** (This is not always easy, but it is a very important reminder.)

**"Begin to listen to what you say. Don't say anything that you don't want to become true for you." — Louise L. Hay** (Before my fibro crash, I never realized how hard I was on myself through my self-talk.)

**"You can't stop the waves, but you can learn to surf." —Jon Kabat-Zinn** (Learning to go with the flow is vital in recovering from FMS/CFS.)

**"Always go with the choice that scares you the most, because that's the one that is going to require the most from you." —Caroline Myss** (The unknown when beginning the Guaifenesin Protocol really scared me, but I knew that I had to take the risk. I am now so thankful that I did.)

**"Look at your life as your main career and your divine classroom." —Judith Orloff** (When I had to resign from my job, this quote helped me move forward.)

**"Do not wait; the time will never be just right. Start where you stand and work with whatever tools you have at your command and better tools will be found as you go along."—George Herbert** (This quote is another motto that I live by to this day. All the way through my FMS/CFS reversal process, whenever I would start to feel afraid or worried, I would recite this to myself.)

**"I am okay." —Chantal K. Hoey-Sanders** (I recite this to myself anytime I start to feel anxious or overwhelmed. Okay, it was about every five minutes during my first year of illness!)

**"I am safe, healthy, vibrant, and strong." —Chantal K. Hoey-Sanders** (I repeat this affirmation whenever I feel the need, as often as I like. Usually I use it when I am approaching a new situation and I am beginning to feel overwhelmed.)

**"I am that I am." — (Exodus 3:14)** (Need I say more? I remind myself of this when I am frustrated that I can't do as much as I used to be able to do prior to my fibromyalgia crash.)

**"When you know better, you do better." —Maya Angelou** (This quote helped me deal with ignorant people and unhelpful doctors.)

**"What we focus our attention on grows, and I chose peace/health rather than this." —Author Unknown** (I recite this daily or when I am feeling anger sneak in.)

**"You must be the change you wish to see in the world." —Mahatama Gandhi** (This quote embodies the Guaifenesin Protocol for me and helps me stay focused and on track with my hypoglycemic diet and joy of movement exercise goals.)

**"We must be willing to get rid of the life that we've planned, so as to accept the life that is waiting for us." —Joseph Campbell** (This quote embodies my fibromyalgia/chronic fatigue experience.)

**"And the day came when the risk it took to remain tight in a bud was more painful than the risk it took to blossom." —Anais Nin** (This quote helped me to overcome my fears and doubts about doing the Guaifenesin Protocol, and it also helped me with applying for disability.)

**"The years teach us much which the days never knew." —Ralph Waldo Emerson** (I apply this to my symptom journal, and it is the best symptom journal advice for reversing my fibromyalgia with Guaifenesin that I have ever received. Hang in there! Three steps forward and two steps back.)

**"The past has no power to keep you from being present now." —Eckhart Tolle, author and spiritual teacher** (Awesome, awesome, awesome! I apply this to every aspect of my life on a daily basis.)

**"Acknowledging the good that is already in your life is the foundation for all abundance." —Eckhart Tolle** (I count my blessings every day, no matter how challenging my day might be.)

**"Dream an even bigger dream." —Oprah Winfrey** (I focused on this quote when wanting and hoping to become pregnant one day.)

**"Life isn't as serious as you make it out to be." —Eckhart Tolle** (Isn't this statement true? It makes me laugh at myself when I read it, because I am always ever so serious.)

**"I can't save you. You have to save yourself." —Jillian Michaels, trainer, *The Biggest Loser*** (Absolutely true. This quote hit me like a ton of bricks and resonated inside of me. I use it in all aspects of the Guaifenesin Protocol, not just the diet.)

**"Believe in yourself. Trust the process. Change forever." —Bob Harper, trainer, *The Biggest Loser*** (Trusting the process was huge for me when I first began the Guai and then later with the HG diet the second time I started on the strict side post-partum when trying to lose my baby weight.)

I have drawn strength from these affirmations over the years while reversing my fibromyalgia with the Guaifenesin Protocol. Countless hours were spent in isolation, trying to relieve myself from some of my suffering by focusing on getting well and utilizing these statements. It's important to say these affirmations over and over again to yourself, even if you don't believe in them or you think that they will not work. Scientific research has proven that we can create perfect health by our thinking; you need to ask yourself what type of health you would like to manifest. (I am no way suggesting here that FMS/CFS is in our heads. Absolutely not! However, as someone who has always been very critical of myself, this shift away from negative thinking has really transformed me. I am living the results of focusing on the positives in life, my life, and I am happy despite my FMS/CFS.)

So remember that you are not this illness. You are not your job or the number on your paycheck. These things don't define who you are as a person, who you *truly* are. And you will get better in time. This is just a bump in the road, your road. This is a short time in the rest of your life, so change your thoughts. You deserve perfect health.

I must add that I have had fun collecting these quotes throughout my years of recovery. It's a hobby that I have created for myself. Before my illness, I never gave quotes a thought. Then suddenly, once I became ill, they would appear in all different situations and I would just jot them down. Maya Angelou's quote was the first one I ever encountered, on the first day after my fibromyalgia crash. One day, as I was waiting to pick up a prescription at the pharmacy (struggling to muster up enough energy to stand there), I happened to stumble across it on a greeting card. I liked the bright orange day lily on the cover, and it caught my attention. The words matched how I was feeling at that very moment, and I clung to them. I needed hope, as I was feeling quite reduced as a human being. I bought the card and used it as my new mantra.

I can't stress enough—and I will repeat this again—how important it is to take the time that you need to grieve what you have lost, but don't get stuck in it. Remember that you are not your illness. Never give it the power to define you. *You may have fibromyalgia, but it doesn't have you!* Find ways to have fun, despite your pain and fatigue, and try to create the person you wish to one day become. Envision yourself healthy, well again, and leading the life of your dreams. In time, you will be able to reflect with a smile.

You won't miss the person or the life you left behind. In fact, you will be amazed at how you respect and cherish this new you!

## Letting Go of Ego: I Am Not My Illness

One day, I got the bright idea to pretend that I was in kindergarten again. For some strange reason, I guess, lying on my futon mattress on the living room floor, debilitated day after day, reminded me of the good old days of naptime in kindergarten. Although I was plagued with pain and fatigue, as silly as it sounds, I gave myself permission to become five years old again, free of responsibilities and stress. I let go of my ego, and in that moment, I realized that I was not my illness. Rather than continuing with my frustration of being sick and what I no longer was able to do, I learned to enjoy the silence and to see my world in a different light.

I began to notice and to relish in the simple things, like the soft purr of my cat and the texture of my blankets and how soft and comforting they felt around my neck. I imagined in my most pain-filled moments that I had four Himalayan kittens tucked in bed with me under my covers, just below my chin, purring away.

Pre-fibromyalgia crash, I had always been very mechanical and able to fix things. If the VCR was broken, I could take it apart and figure out why. Not anymore. My ability to follow and read simple directions was gone. I could not remember how to do simple things like turn the water off in the bathtub or unload the dishwasher. My brain was completely jumbled. The migraine pain and bodily fatigue had taken over. I was completely frustrated at first, and my ego was bent out of shape. I had to re-teach myself how to do everything. This was embarrassing and humiliating. But rather than letting my negative self-thoughts destroy me, I decided to shift my self-thinking. I said good-bye to my ego, and I never once let this illness define me. Again, I believed, "I am not fibromyalgia. I have fibromyalgia, but it doesn't have me!"

Here are a couple of my posts from the GuaiGroup, an online forum *(www.fibromyalgiatreatment.com)* run by Claudia Craig Marek, co-author of *What Your Doctor May Not Tell You about Fibromyalgia.*

> Hello Fellow Guaier!
>
> I wanted to respond to your post.
>
> After being completely misunderstood by everyone in my life and bedridden—on a futon mattress in the middle of

my living room floor in the dark for months—because I was too weak to walk upstairs to my bed—in too much pain to move—with a migraine that lasted for years—what I learned to do that helped me were a couple of things—

First—try not to expect people (normals) to understand. When you do find someone who does understand you and wants to learn more about your condition really cherish them. I found that the less I expected of myself and others around me the better I felt.

Next—since I was bedridden and unable to go to work, to read, to watch television, or get dressed—I really felt like a failure. So, what I began to do was imagine that I was in another place—a safe place. Although I consciously knew that I was on the mattress in the middle of my living room floor in so much pain that I couldn't move—I changed my thoughts. I put myself in another place. In my mind I was floating on the water on one of those inflatable mattresses on a lake in the mountains at dusk. My mattress was attached to a dock so I wouldn't worry about drifting off too far. I used this technique along with deep abdominal breathing exercises when ever and where ever my pain or anxiety got to be too much and it did help me. In fact, it was the only thing that kept me moving forward until I found acupuncture, soft tissue manipulation, the strict HG diet, and of course, Guaifenesin.

Try to change—and this is challenging—every negative thought that you have—about yourself, about others, about being sick— into a positive one. Instead of thinking—I am so sick. I am never going to get better. Say to yourself—I am so sick now, BUT I am on my way to great health! Then change that thought to—I can feel great health, I am creating my own great health every day. I am getting healthier everyday! The Guaifenesin is working. I AM making it work! The more we do this the more we do create our own great health and empower ourselves. You will have your rough days, but you will get better in time.

Being sick and then getting well, is a process and a journey and you will get there. You will. We all will. So, try to look at the "positives of being sick"—they are there even though you may not notice them now. Let yourself be angry at the illness and then channel that anger into getting well. You can do it!

Hello Fellow Guaier,

You are not alone. I have been where you are now and it's not fun, but it will get better. You will get better!

Normals simply don't understand this illness so rather than to waste all your energy on trying to make them understand, you have to change your focus. You had mentioned that you have a cat. Try to focus—on something positive— like on your cat's purr and the fact that your cat loves you just the way you are. And, he or she is really happy to be able to snuggle with you right now.

Whenever you get really down "see" yourself doing something that you love to do and that you one day will be able to do again. If your pain is too great—practice relaxation techniques and deep abdominal breathing. Focus on a safe place in your mind—a place where you are at peace and out of pain. Imagine yourself well again. (Here is an excerpt from my fibro journal on how to imagine yourself well again.)

### **Three Years Later on** Guaifenesin **and AFTER the MOVE to a new City**

"Hi Kitties," I say, as I enter my bedroom. They know the daily drill. I am flat on my back, on my unmade bed, in between my kitties. I meditate and breathe. Clear my mind for a few seconds. In my mind I picture myself well. I see myself doing what I will be doing today. I mentally walk myself through it. I rehearse it and practice it in my mind. In my mind, I am successful.

I yawn and stretch. I place a hand on each kitty. They are like two warm and fluffy soft motors welcoming me onto the bed. They don't mind that I am partially dressed with semi-dried hair, no make-up and sunglasses. Their purring comforts me—assures me that I am okay in the moment. A third kitty enters the room. He is the grand daddy of them all. Mitch is fourteen years old, black and white with the loudest most soothing purr. He needs help getting on to the bed. I help him up. I understand his struggle.

Each day as I go through this wake-up get dressed ritual, I practice and I remind myself of how far I have come. I focus on my breath. I praise myself for the fact that I am no longer bedridden. I honor my being by my gentle way with myself. I cherish those kitties who have seen me through. I thank God and the universe for allowing me this experience. I wish for continued improvements and great health. I realize that I am in control of my thoughts and that my possibilities are endless. I hope this helps you.

Chantal in Michigan

# Part 4

## Reversing Fibromyalgia with Guaifenesin

# Chapter 4:
# The Fourth Step: Realizing Hope Is Here

"You deserve perfect. You have already done old age [with your fibromyalgia]. Now it is time for youthing."

—R. Paul St. Amand, MD

I am fortunate. Although I know I don't need a local doctor to follow the Guaifenesin Treatment Protocol, I do have one who is willing to help me restore my health and reverse this dreadful disease. Incredibly, he understands how very ill I am and he believes wholeheartedly in Dr. St. Amand's work. I am very grateful that he has taken me under his wing. Even though I am only his second patient on the protocol, he is confident that I will get well. He told me, "This is a learning process. We will work together. We will both acquire knowledge about the Guaifenesin Protocol together. Although I am the doctor, you too will become my teacher."

We begin. Dr. Struwa follows Dr. St. Amand's lead by making sure that I have had all blood tests to rule out other medical conditions that may mimic fibromyalgia or may be in addition to my fibromyalgia. We discuss the laboratory results and tests that I have already had done. We get everything in order and ready for me to start the Guaifenesin.

If you are interested in beginning the Guaifenesin Protocol, it is imperative that you first receive an official diagnosis of fibromyalgia by a licensed medical practitioner and have the appropriate blood work and medical tests done to rule out more serious medical conditions. You don't necessarily need a specialist to make the correct diagnosis. General practitioners or internists are perfectly qualified to help you. Make sure, however, that you find a doctor who actually believes that fibromyalgia exists. Call around and ask the secretary before you schedule your appointment. It may sound silly to take this precaution, but it can save you time, money, wasted energy, and the frustration of not being heard or understood.

Since fibromyalgia affects every cell in my body, every doctor that I work with now must be familiar with it and trust its existence. I actually schedule an "appointment interview" beforehand with all of my doctors from ophthalmologist to gynecologist and make sure that they believe fibromyalgia is real. If they don't, I don't become their patient.

Your next step in beginning the Guaifenesin Protocol requires you to purchase or borrow from your local library the 2006 copyrighted revised and updated version of the book, *What Your Doctor May Not Tell You about Fibromyalgia.* You may buy the book from *www.amazon.com, www.barnesandnoble.com,* or *www.fibromyalgiatreatment.com.* Please keep in mind that all proceeds from the last website go to support Dr. St. Amand's research. This book also has a free online support group called the Guai Group that you may join if you so choose.

The following account does not replace the advice of a medical doctor; rather, it is an introduction to a new treatment option that might be right for you.

## Ruling Out Other Medical Conditions

Dr. St. Amand recommends that a basic work up should be ordered. Fasting samples should also be drawn. A blood count looking for anemia, infection, or inflammation is recommended. A chemistry panel will look at your liver and your kidneys, screen for lipid abnormalities, diabetes, and the chemical composition of your serum. Remember that a normal blood sugar level does not exclude hypoglycemia and a low sugar blood fasting level demands further investigation possibly by an endocrinologist. The outstandingly accurate thyroid test of TSH (thyroid stimulating hormone) is mandatory for the detection of glandular dysfunction. It's very common for hypothyroidism and fibromyalgia often times to overlap just by chance and each condition will make the other one worse. Your doctor may want to test for Lyme's Disease or other locally occurring possibilities. A liver test might be ordered to test for hepatitis if you have traveled extensively. Depending on your age, other possibilities exist. Your doctor may include an arthritis panel in the blood tests. If you are over fifty and a woman you should be tested for polymyalgia rheumatica using the ESR (erythrocyte sedimentation rate.) Make sure that you bring a complete list of all of your medications and supplements that you are taking as some of these can alter liver enzymes and kidney function. Since there are no distinguishing tests at this time to rule out fibromyalgia, the work being ordered on your blood is to reassure you that and your physician that something more urgent doesn't exist or co-exist with your fibromyalgia.

The diagnosis of fibromyalgia is made in two parts. In the first part, the doctor will take a detailed medical history that includes a full systems review. The second part consists of a hands-on search for the so-called tender points. Make sure that they examine the other areas that hurt, even if they are not part of the predetermined ones.

I had been diagnosed previously with migraines, anxiety, irritable bowel syndrome, irritable bladder, acid reflux, and polycystic ovarian disease with hirsutism (excess bodily hair, mostly on the face). Polycystic ovarian disease and hirsutism are not related to fibromyalgia. For years, I had suffered with many other bodily complaints that were never fully addressed because none of my doctors was able to link all of them together and see the bigger fibromyalgia/chronic fatigue picture. This continued for me until age thirty-two, when I met Dr. Srutwa, my local MD acupuncturist, and I got lucky.

An emergency room doctor for twenty-two years, Dr. Srtuwa recognized right away that I had fibromyalgia/chronic fatigue syndrome. He could feel my "painful hard places" or "lumps and bumps" as I called them. Since he specialized in the muscles, he immediately did a hands-on examination by feeling my muscles in two-inch increments and identifying my tender points or trigger points, as used to describe myofascial pain. (For more information about myofascial pain and fibromyalgia, please visit *www.*sover.net/~devstar/.) None of my other doctors had done that before.

Currently, the official American College of Rheumatology (ACR) criteria for the diagnosis of fibromyalgia, established in 1990, states that patients must have widespread pain in four quadrants of their body for a minimum duration of three months and experience moderate pain and tenderness at a minimum of eleven out of eighteen predetermined sites or tender points when appropriate pressure is exerted by an examiner. However, as of press time, the American College of Rheumatology (ACR) (*www.rheumatology.org*) is proposing new diagnostic criteria for fibromyalgia that includes common symptoms such as fatigue, sleep problems, as well as cognitive problems and pain. The tender-point test is being replaced with a widespread pain index and a symptom severity scale.

In his office, Dr. Srutwa explained the importance of this to me. He told me that he stopped counting my tender points once he had reached forty-five. We both chuckled and found the humor in it, although it wasn't very funny. Needless to say, I was in extreme pain. Normally the diagnosis of fibromyalgia is made with *eleven* out of *eighteen* predetermined tender points. He stopped counting my tender points at forty-five!

Absolutely, I was ready to begin the Guaifenesin Treatment Protocol and reverse this dreadful syndrome. Dr. Srutwa and I further discussed the Guaifenesin Protocol, how the Guaifenesin works in its reversal process, and its other vital components, including the hypoglycemia diet (if blood sugar issues are apparent and you are hypoglycemic), the Guaifenesin, the salicylates, the symptom journal, and the mapping.

Since I have been following the hypoglycemic diet perfectly for two months now, much of my cognitive function has been restored. I am able to read, to comprehend, and to retain information again. It is wonderful and I feel empowered. It's time for me to tackle the salicylates: Guaifenesin's main blocker and enemy.

## Using Guaifenesin to Reverse Fibromyalgia/Chronic Fatigue Syndrome

Guaifenesin is an expectorant that thins mucus and helps to loosen phlegm. Guaifenesin is quickly absorbed from the gastrointestinal tract, and is rapidly metabolized and excreted in the urine. It is also known to lower uric acid levels. No serious side effects have been reported. It is now available over the counter.

## Summarizing Dr. St. Amand's Theory of Fibromyalgia/Chronic Fatigue Syndrome

(Quoted and reproduced with permission from the authors *www.fibromyalgiatreatment.com.*)

Here is a copy of Dr. St. Amand's theory of fibromyalgia, how he maps his patients and uses Guaifenesin and avoids salicylates to reverse the illness. (I have included a copy of an example of a typical fibromyalgia map, with its marked tender points at the back of this book.)

## The Guaifenesin Protocol for the Treatment of Fibromyalgia

by R. Paul St. Amand, MD

## FIBROMYALGIA

*Fibromyalgia is a cyclic and a symptomatically progressive illness that affects millions of people regardless of race. It is manifested by many complaints that initially last only a few days, but are later unrelenting. Recurrent attacks eventually involve multiple body areas and systems until patients simply cycle from bad to worse. Patients are typically referred from doctor to doctor based on individual complaints. The partially-informed professional may fail to grasp the extent of the problem and divide the disease into symptom-packages that lead to medical dead ends such as chronic fatigue, systemic candidiasis, myofascial pain, irritable bowel, or vulvar pain syndrome. There are no diagnostic x-ray or laboratory tests for fibromyalgia.*

*The American College of Rheumatology recommends eliciting pain from at least eleven sites from eighteen predetermined "tender points" to confirm the diagnosis. Unfortunately, individual pain perception and tenderness vary greatly. So-called chronic fatigue patients have high pain thresholds and are not particularly sensitive to finger-poking. They may feel stiff, but complain mainly of fatigue and cognitive impairment. We urge physicians to seek objective evidence and stop relying on purely subjective responses. The confirmation of fibromyalgia is more reliably obtained by using our method of palpation that we call mapping (see below).*

*Fibromyalgia has no set symptoms. Various combinations from the following list can be anticipated:*

***Central Nervous System:*** *Fatigue, irritability, nervousness, depression, apathy, listlessness, impaired memory and concentration, anxieties and even suicidal thoughts. Insomnia and frequent awakening due to pain result in non restorative sleep.*

***Musculoskeletal:*** *Swollen structures press on nerves to produce all types of pains especially morning stiffness. Any muscle, tendon, ligament or fascia in the face, neck, shoulders, back, hips, knees, ankles, feet, arms, legs and chest may participate. They also cause calf/foot cramps, numbness and tingling of the face or extremities. Old, injured, or operative sites are commonly affected. Fibromyalgia is erroneously considered non-arthritic even though joint pain, swelling, heat and redness are common.*

***Irritable Bowel:*** *(Often called leaky gut, spastic colon, or mucous colitis). Symptoms include nausea (usually transient, repetitive waves), indigestion, gas, bloating, deep pain, cramps, alternating constipation and diarrhea sometimes with mucous stools.*

***Genitourinary:*** *Mostly affecting women are pungent urine, frequent urination, bladder spasms, burning urination (dysuria) with or without repeated bladder infections and interstitial cystitis. Vulvodynia (vulvar pain syndrome) includes vaginal spasm, irritation of the labia (vulvitis) or deeper (vestibulitis) that induce painful intercourse (dyspareunia) all without the typical cottage-cheese discharge that accompanies yeast infections. Fibromyalgia is worse premenstrually as are PMS and uterine cramping.*

***Dermatological:*** *Various rashes may appear with or without itching: Hives, red blotches, itchy bumps or blisters, eczema, seborrheic or neurodermatitis, and rosacea. Skin is dry and nails are brittle or easily peel; hair is of poor quality and often falls out prematurely. Strange sensations (paresthesias) are common such as cold, burning (especially palms, soles and thighs), crawling, electric vibrations, prickling, super-sensitivity to touch, and flushing often with sweating.*

***Head, Eye, Ear, Nose, and Throat:*** *Headaches (migraines), dizziness, vertigo (spinning) or imbalance; itchy, burning and dry eyes or lids sometimes produce morning sticky or sandy discharges; blurred vision; hay fever or nasal congestion and post-nasal drip; painful, burning or cut-tongue sensation, scalded mouth and abnormal tastes (bad, metallic); intermittent low-pitched sounds or transient ringing in the ears (tinnitus); ear and eyeball pain; sensitivity to light, sounds and odors (perfumes or chemicals).*

***Miscellaneous Symptoms:*** *Weight gain; mild fever; reduced immunity to infection; fluid retention with morning eyelid and hand swelling that gravitates to the legs by evening, stretches tiny tissue nerves to produce restless leg syndrome; adult-onset asthma.*

***Hypoglycemia Syndrome:*** *This is a separate entity that may affect thirty percent of female and fifteen percent of male fibromyalgics fibroglycemia). Sugar craving, tremors, clamminess, anxiety, panic attacks, heart pounding, headaches and faintness induced by hunger or by eating sugar and starches (carbohydrates) are solid clues for diagnosis. Hypoglycemics must follow a prescribed diet or they will not fully reverse symptoms that strongly overlap those of fibromyalgia.*

*Though fibromyalgia is almost always inherited, injury, infection surgery, and stress may prod susceptible individuals into overt attacks. We have seen patients as young as age two as well as presenting in the seventies. Family histories often span three and four generations. Boys and girls are equally affected before puberty, but in adults, females heavily predominate (85 percent). Forty-five percent of adults remember growing pains in childhood that disappeared with the growth spurt of puberty. If untreated, we believe fibromyalgia evolves into a tartar of joints and the eventual damage of osteoarthritis.*

*Forty-seven years ago, a man taking a gout medication noticed he could peel calculus (a calcium phosphate compound) off his teeth with his fingernail. This mundane observation raised the possibility that tartar was a reflection of an unrecognized systemic problem expressed in saliva. I postulated a genetically defective enzyme prominent in the kidney that would cause a backup of phosphate throughout the system. Excesses of this ion in certain cell structures (mitochondria) would seriously impede the formation of energy (ATP). The resulting cellular fatigue would cause wide-spread malfunctions that would easily explain all the symptoms of fibromyalgia. Our paper for interested professionals defends that theory.*

*We treat fibromyalgia using Guaifenesin. It increases urinary excretion of phosphate, gradually extracts abnormal body-wide accumulations, and thus reverses the illness. Guaifenesin is devoid of significant side effects and totally safe for children. It has been marketed for over fifty years for loosening and increasing the flow of mucus. Manufacturing processes seem to determine its potency, effectiveness and duration of action. We monitor and recommend the brands that have proven adequate for our purposes. Excessively short-acting tablets lack twenty-four hour action. Combination long-short formulations may fail due to insufficient contents of either component. We determine what works for individuals by sequential physical examinations (next paragraph). Treatment is begun using reliable products at 300 mg twice daily for the first week. The drug has no significant side effects so that worsening symptoms suggests that is the correct dosage for reversal, an amount that works for only 20% of patients. If there are no significant changes that first week, we raise the dosage to 600 mg. twice daily and hold there until the next examination. The response rate at this amount is 80%. Obviously, 20% of patients will need further adjustments. We repeat the muscle examination monthly (see below) until sufficient areas disappear to confirm the adequacy of dosage. Symptoms frequently intensify during the clearing process and new ones may surface due to increased intensity. This confirms that purging is underway because* Guaifenesin *has no side effects. Better hours eventually cluster into days and finally weeks. During this process, lesions objectively soften upon examination, sometimes split, and gradually vanish. Recovery is rapid compared to the time it took to develop the illness. Even the slowest responders clear at least one year's accumulated debris every two months. The earliest lesions are the last to clear.*

*The original description of fibromyalgia as "rheumatism with hard and tender places" has been forgotten. The often-recommended tender-point exam seeks subjective patient pain sensations from eighteen predetermined areas. It is of limited value compared to objective, sequential body examinations (mapping) that help establish the dosage and document disease reversal. We examine musculoskeletal tissues using the pads of our fingers to feel muscles, tendons, and ligaments. With practice, multiple swollen places become obvious. We sketch their location, size and degree of hardness on a caricature that becomes our baseline for future comparisons (figure 1). Hands should move as if to iron out wrinkles in the underlying tissues. Expressions of tenderness do not influence findings. The most important site for confirming the diagnosis and establishing the dosage is the left thigh. The outside of the quadriceps muscle (Vastus lateralis) and the front part (Rectus femoris) are involved in 100% of adults; they clear within the first month of proper treatment.*

*To ignore the following guarantees failure: aspirin and other sources of salicylate block the action of* Guaifenesin *at the same kidney level as they do other uricosuric medications. A person's genetic makeup determines susceptibility to blocking. Nevertheless to assure success, everyone should adhere to the protocol and make no modifications. Salicylates are present in many pain medications such as aspirin and those for some forms of colitis. Salicylate is absorbed through intact skin as well as the thin membranes of the mouth and intestine. Products used topically or as medications should be inspected for ingredients including all synthetic forms such as octisalate in sunscreens and wintergreen in gum. Almost all plant species have substantial levels of the natural chemical. Quantities vary from crop to crop and are stored to fend off infections and to help heal injuries. For this reason herbal medications block* Guaifenesin *as do plant extracts and oils including camphor.*

*The following is an incomplete guide to sources of natural and synthetic salicylates:*

***MEDICATIONS:*** *(1.) Pain relievers containing salicylate or salicylic acid, for example, aspirin, Salflex, Anacin, Excedrin, Disalcid. (2.) Herbal medications such as St. John's Wort, gingko biloba, saw palmetto, evening primrose oil, Echinacea. Vitamins with rose hips, bioflavonoids (quercetin, hesperiden or rutin) or plant extracts such as alfalfa. (3.) Some wart or callus removers, acne products and dandruff shampoos contain salicylic acid. (4.) Topical pain creams such as Tiger Balm, Ben Gay, Myoflex.(5.) Medications such as Pepto Bismol, Asacol, Alka Seltzer and Urised.*

***COSMETIC AND TOPICAL PRODUCTS*** *(1.) Skin cleansers (exfoliants) that use salicylic acid or witch hazel. (2.) Hair products with plant extracts such as balsam or bisabol. (3.) Bubble baths with essential oils such as lavender. (4.) Watch for the letters "SAL" in sunscreens: octisalate, homosalate, or the name meradimate or mexoryl. (5.) Lip balms containing camphor or menthol. (6.) Lipsticks, glosses and deodorants should be checked for castor oil. (7.) When gardening wear waterproof gloves, avoid barefoot contact with freshly cut grass. (8.) Avoid tissue or wipes containing aloe. (9.) Shaving creams with aloe or menthol will block. (10.) Do not use razors with aloe strips (Vitamin E, lanolin, and baby Oil are acceptable.) (11.) Moisturizers with oils such as almond, extracts such as green tea, or gels such as arnica.*

***ORAL AGENTS:*** *(1.) Most mouth washes contain mint, wintergreen or salicylate (Listerine). (2.) Toothpastes contain salicylates, as well as fresh or synthetic mint, often unlisted. Use non mint toothpastes made by Tom's of Maine, Cleure or Personal Basics. Baking soda and/or peroxide also provide good cleansing and whitening. The non-mint pre-brushing rinses are acceptable as are the Cleure mouthwashes; (3.) Avoid lozenges, floss, breath fresheners or chewing gum with mint flavor (menthol, wintergreen, peppermint or spearmint). (Strong fruit and/Cinnamon flavors may mask unlisted mint)*

***YOU MUST TAKE RESPONSIBILITY FOR THE PROTOCOL. PHYSICIANS ARE NOT TRAINED TO RECOGNIZE SALICYLATE-CONTAINING INGREDIENTS.*** *If you fail, you will convince your doctor* Guaifenesin *does not work and the opportunity to help other fibromyalgics will be lost. Dictionaries can help you identify ingredients. Get the full list of contents when you phone manufacturers because customer service employees will not know that plants make salicylates. Our website* www.fibromyalgiatreatment.com *connects you with a knowledgeable support group that will help you with questions. The site* www.fibromyalgiatreatment.com/board *keeps updated listings of safe products and new information.*

*No diet is required for fibromyalgia because the liver has a certain but limited capacity to counter food salicylates. It cannot override excesses from plant concentrates obtained from juicing or in herbal medications. Teas are high in salicylate and should be used sparingly.*

*Decongestants and cough medicines have side effects and should not be used as sources for Guaifenesin. Pure* Guaifenesin *has no side effects (rarely transient nausea) and no known drug interactions. Pain medications such as acetaminophen (Tylenol), Ultram, Darvocet-N, Imitrex, and non-steroidal drugs such as Advil and Aleve, do not block Guaifenesin. Especially when dealing with chronic illness, we chose not to prescribe narcotics such as codeine, hydrocodone (Vicodin), oxycontin, morphine, or methadone even though they are not blockers. They are too liberally prescribed for pain control at the price of eventual addiction. When our mapping indicates it is time to discontinue them, intense withdrawal effects usually occur. All too many patients fail in the attempt since, as the drug wears off; the brain reproduces identical symptoms that once originated in outlying tissues.*

*Our treatment is not for the faint of heart. It demands a patient's skill and determination with or without professional supervision. Remember, reversal of the disease reproduces past symptoms and can induce new ones. We repeat they are not side effects. Though the intensity of the early reversal may cause concern it is similar to a rollercoaster ride that gets progressively tamer. We offer hope to those with willpower to try once again despite previous failures. Meticulously done, this is a highly-effective protocol.*

This condensed version of the Guaifenesin Protocol really struck a positive chord inside of me. I can completely relate to it. It is my story. I am ready. It's time that I expand and I buy my own copy of the book. I want to be able to write in it and take notes in its margins. Yes, this book is my new "Fibromyalgia bible," and it's now imperative that I have my own copy. Dr. Srutwa has been kind enough to lend me one of his copies, but now that I am beginning to read again, it is mandatory that I get my own.

I know that I am going to get well. I feel it. I am not sure about the exact time frame, and that is okay. Dr. St. Amand states that we clear one year of illness for every two months correctly on the protocol. Although I do have many concerns about how my body will react to the Guaifenesin, I realize that these concerns are okay. I will not let fear hold me back from my recovery.

Together Dr. Srutwa and I are gradually learning about the protocol. Although I know I do not need a local doctor to help me reverse on the Guaifenesin Protocol, I do need the weekly support and pain management. This means that I will need to schedule my weekly office visits with him in advance.

Dr. Srutwa believes in me, and little by little, I am beginning to believe in myself once again. I can do this! Encouraged, I leave his office with a sincere hope for the first time in almost a year.

My Thursday mornings suddenly remind me of the book, *Tuesdays with Morrie*, and they quickly become my Thursdays with Thaddeus, although he is always very respectfully Dr. Srutwa to me. I sign up for a two-hour session with him for soft-tissue manipulation, myofascial pain release, trigger-point injections, and acupuncture with electrical stimulation.

I register myself for more therapies. I know that as a human being, I am multi-dimensional mind, body, and spirit, with all three being closely intertwined and that I will benefit from other healing modalities, as long as they don't block the Guaifenesin.

In the course of the next year, I try cranial-sacral work, reflexology, physical therapy, the foot bath, homeopathic remedies, tai chi home stretches, and chiropractic adjustments with the activator machine. I commit to several consecutive treatments in order to give them a chance. I continue checking out more books on tape from my local library and learn more about guided imagery, visualization, and meditation. I believe that each of these therapies has its own perfect place in my healing and wellness. I join the online support group GuaiGroup *(www.fibromyalgiatreatment.com)* and become a lurker. I secretly read and study the list serve message board and gather as much information about the protocol as my fibro-fogged brain can withstand. One day, I plan on introducing myself to this group, but not quite yet.

I continue with the physical therapy exercises, reflexology, trigger-point injections, soft-tissue manipulation, acupuncture, and tai chi home stretches. I feel these have helped me the most. I become a faithful daily lurker on the GuaiGroup forums. I am making the strict HG diet work for me. I keep my pre-scheduled 11 AM Thursday appointments with Dr. Srutwa, even though I am not a morning person. We discuss the Guaifenesin Protocol at each meeting, he maps me, I keep a detailed symptom journal, and every Thursday morning for the next three years, with his guidance and encouragement, I am beyond hopeful.

I have followed the HG strict diet perfectly for more than two months now. At each visit, we talk about my home life and my symptoms. Dr. Srutwa notices that my fibro-fog has improved and that I am losing weight. He asks me about my sleep history. I tell him that it is variable and that although I am on the strict hypoglycemic diet, the fact still remains that I am having trouble falling asleep and I never feel rested in the morning when I get up. This has been a great problem of mine for years.

Truth be told, I have been an insomniac since I was about fifteen years old. Frequent urination all night is one of my most annoying symptoms, although I am not a diabetic. We decide that I need to eat a piece of cheese when I awaken at three in the morning, as recommended by Dr. St. Amand. This will aid in stabilizing my blood sugar and help me get back to sleep. I am carbohydrate intolerant. This slice of cheese that I now eat in the middle of the night does help me with my urgency to go to the bathroom and I no longer have my night sweats, and this is more than wonderful. Again, who would have thought that food could change my body like this for the better and so drastically?

You must address the possibility of being hypoglycemic (or as Dr. St. Amand describes it in great detail in chapter 5 of his book, the condition he coined *fibroglycemic*). Neither the glucose tolerance test, nor the fasting blood sugar test for diabetes will accurately determine if you are hypoglycemic. The only way that you will know is by monitoring your symptoms, trying the diet, and seeing how you react to it. The more you crave sugars, the more you need to avoid them. The sicker you feel the first two weeks on the hypoglycemic diet, the more your body really needs it. This is your body's natural way of adjusting to it. I know it sounds surreal, but it is true. Trust me.

It is now Thursday morning. Dr. Srutwa feels that my inability to sleep is contributing to my lingering fibro-fog, and he would like me to try Ambien. I agree to try it.

Another week passes and although I am still *not* feeling well rested in the mornings when I wake up, the Ambien has actually helped me fall asleep at night and the cheese slice that I eat at around three o'clock in the morning puts me back to sleep. I consider this fantastic. I am making slow and steady progress. I tell myself, "Baby steps, Chantal, baby steps. Fibromyalgia is a complex syndrome, and for every three steps you take forward, you will also be taking two steps backward in your reversal process with the Guaifenesin—and that is okay."

The following Thursday, after reviewing my sleep history for the week, Dr. Srutwa recommended that I try Flexeril for my muscles for sleep. He reasoned that the stiffness of my muscles and the pain that this generates at night while lying down can also be keeping me awake all night. Although I am not fond of medications, I had been on thirteen at one point after my initial Mayo Clinic visit, I agreed to try this new medication. I believe that anything that can aid me in my recovery while on the Guaifenesin Protocol, as long as it doesn't block the Guaifenesin, deserves a chance. That night I took the two pills at bedtime, and I noticed that they helped me immediately.

We continued to talk more about my home life, and I realized that I did need to cut myself some slack. I felt guilty not being able to go to work or do housework. I missed the teaching life that I had left behind.

Dr. Srtuwa's undergraduate degree was in psychology—how very fortunate for me. He very gently reminded me that getting well isn't only about learning how to do the mechanical aspects of the Guaifenesin Protocol or the logistics of changing my lifestyle of eating. It's also about learning how to be kind to myself while I am doing it. "You need to learn to love yourself, Chantal," he explained. I was at first taken aback by his statement, and I felt that it was rather corny. In fact, I left his office wondering what kind of a doctor makes a statement like that to his patients.

I reflected on his comment on my short drive home and realized, somewhere deep inside of me, that he was right. I felt that it was true. I did need to learn how to love myself. I have always been too hard on myself. I grew up thinking that the stricter and more diligent I was with myself, the better person I would one day become. Now I am finding that this thinking was actually very negative and damaging to my overall well-being. I am not insinuating that I in any way caused my fibromyalgia. Rather, I am just facing the facts that my wellness will require much work to be done on myself: mind, body, and spirit, and that is okay. "Baby steps, Chantal, baby steps."

## Discovering Movement: Tai Chi and Physical Therapy

Today Dr. Srutwa greeted me in his waiting room and presented me with a paper titled, "Tai Chi Range of Motion Exercises." (I have included a copy in the back of this book.) He told me that it is important that I begin to move again. He understood that it wouldn't be easy. He also introduced me to some simple tai chi stretches that I could do at home and demonstrated how I should do them. I was a bit embarrassed to be moving my stiff and not-so-in-shape body this way, but I quickly got over it.

I am to do them daily. I can break them down into sections if I need to. I can progress at my own pace, but it is essential that I follow them daily. He informed me that my inactivity from being bedridden without a bed on the futon mattress in the middle of our living room floor over the past year had actually made my muscles worse. These exercises will help with my muscle stiffness, while also gradually restoring my energy levels. He reminded me again of Dr. St. Amand's theory that individuals with fibromyalgia can't produce energy properly and that the more I move my body, the more energy I will make and have. I agreed to give them a try. He also wanted me to begin physical therapy, and he gave me the name of a therapist to contact. My life is certainly progressing quickly.

We moved on and discussed my diet. I am to remain on the strict side for more weight loss. In preparation for beginning the Guaifenesin, I am to start tackling the salicylates in my products. I need to learn more about salicylates and how they will block the action of Guaifenesin. Removing the salicylates from my life is a must for ensuring my success on the protocol, and there was no way around it.

Once I left his office, I realized how overwhelmed I have been feeling. Tackling the salicylates feels almost unmanageable, but I know that I can do it. I will find someone who can help me. I will break it down into parts. Collect my products little by little. Pace myself. I will ask for help. I will take the time that I need to study and learn more about the salicylates. I will visit the GuaiGroup website and lurk for a while.

I do understand Dr. St. Amand's theory behind the protocol, and I do believe it will work. I am already experiencing great improvements with just the diet alone. Now it is time to go through all of my personal body products like deodorant, shampoo, and cosmetics, and figure out which ones to donate. I am determined. I will make this protocol work. I won't let my fears or doubts get the best of me. I am committed. I can do this!

## Ensuring Success by Eliminating Salicylates

Salicylic acid is a hormone produced by plants naturally as a protective agent against soil bacteria. Without salicylates, plants would never get off the ground alive. Plants with high salicylate content have been around since 1500 BC. Aspirin is now made synthetically and naturally, therefore, found in many products. It completely blocks the effectiveness of Guaifenesin at the kidney level (St. Amand and Marek 2006, pp. 72–97).

I am not sure that I understand this definition. Okay, I guess it means that I need to avoid aspirin and all the medications I take and topicals on the skin that contain aspirin. But since all plants naturally produce salicylic acid to protect themselves against soil bacteria, that means that I need to avoid anything natural found in the form of gels, oils, or extracts. In his book, Dr. St. Amand states that I need to take responsibility for the protocol for myself and that I need to figure out which of my personal body products like deodorant and shampoo contain salicylates. I will start by boxing up all of my products and using the bare minimum. This shouldn't be too difficult. I haven't worn make-up since I became sick. It is just too tiring to put it on. This is my plan: I will check the ingredients on each product label one by one. I will invest in a magnifying glass and look for Latin sounding names and any oils, gels, or extracts because these are usually plants and full of salicylates. Mineral oil and shea butter, however, are both natural but *not* salicylate containing. Sometimes I will see "sal-" written in the word and know immediately that this is my enemy. Any plant, extract, or oil that is found in concentrated amounts or strong enough to improve my health status will block the action of Guaifenesin. I will donate those items that I can no longer use to friends and family members and remove them from my premises to avoid future product confusion.

Mint in any form—menthol, spearmint, peppermint—will be my greatest enemy and biggest Guaifenesin blocker. Oils, sunscreens, and acne medications can have the words "salicylic acid" written in the ingredients too and these will also block me.

Today is Thursday and I am more than ready to go over my products and search for salicylates with Dr. Srutwa. I have actually collected them and brought them in with me. I know that I will feel more confident if I let him have a look. *I am gently reminded that I must take responsibility for the protocol myself. Physicians are not trained to recognize salicylate-containing ingredients.* Dr. Srutwa agreed with me that my products all appeared to be salicylate free. But then he asked me a funny question, "What type of toilet paper and facial tissue do you use?" Next he proceeded to tell me that companies are now putting aloe and chamomile oil in their products and both are salicylates! So I should double check the packaging on tissues and toilet paper. I am to wear waterproof gloves when I garden, and I am never to go barefoot on grass that's just been cut. I should never, ever put any type of oil, gels, or extracts on my skin if they are made from certain plants. I am still allowed to eat olive oil because normal food quantities won't block me. As long as I don't slather olive oil all over my skin, I am safe eating it. But I am also to be cautious and to avoid items in my vitamins such as quercetin and rose hips.

Of course, even in deciphering salicylates, there is always an exception to the rule. Not all parts of all plants produce salicylates. CRROWS is an acronym used to remember Corn, Rice, Rye, Oats, Wheat, and Soy. Any ingredient made from the seeds or grains of corn, rice, rye, oats, wheat, or soy is okay to use. Anything else, made from the stems, leaves, roots, silk, blossom, etc. is not. In other words, you need to avoid all oils, gels and extracts with a plant name *except* if they contain corn, rice, rye, oats, wheat, or soy. These grains do not block the Guaifenesin. But you still have to avoid the plants they grow on (wheat grass, for example, is a blocker, but wheat germ oil isn't).

Toothpaste and anything minty that is readily absorbed in my mouth by my gums will be another one of my biggest blockers, so I will pay special attention and order some of these items—lip balm, mouthwash, and gum—off of the Internet from salicylate-free companies. In fact, I might just order all of my products from these salicylate-free companies until I get this salicylate thing mastered. Yes, these companies do exist. I recommend Personal Basics by Andrea Rose *(www.andrearose.com)*; Paula's Choice *(www.paulaschoice.com)* (use only products marked as salicylate-free); Cleure *(www.cleure.com)*; and Marina del Rey Pharmacy *(www.fibropharmacy.com)*. Here's a big shout-out thank you to our predecessors for making this salicylate searching and product-buying easier for us.) For more information and a complete list of acceptable over-the- counter products for ensuring your success with searching for salicylates, visit *http://www.fibromyalgiatreatment.com/board.*

## Keeping the Symptom Journal and Being Mapped

Now that I am familiar with the salicylates, it is time for me to figure out how I am going to keep my symptom journal. I know that this is going to be the single most important indicator and manner to track my progress. It is the only tangible way to demonstrate my improvements besides going to California and becoming a patient of Dr. St. Amand's and having him or Claudia body map me personally. Although body mapping is recommended, Dr. St. Amand cautions that if a body mapper has not been trained by him, most likely they will not know how to map correctly. The symptom journal will show you patterns over time of the cycling or purging out of the calcium phosphate. It will be your link to determine if you are blocking the Guaifenesin or hindering it from working. It is a must.

I decided to print off a few copies of the Body Map with Symptom Checklist from the Fibromyalgia Treatment Center's website *(www.fibromyalgiatreatment.com)* only to realize after a few days that this system is not going to work for me. My environmentally conscious self does not enjoy using so much paper daily.

At once, the teacher in me takes over and decides to create my own month-at-a-glance daily fibromyalgia symptom list. I use it for a few months but soon realize that I need to find a way to more specifically record my findings. I can try to write the corresponding number of pain levels (1 to 10) in the boxes next to each symptom. After a few days, this quickly becomes too tedious and not exactly what I need. I decide to have Josh see if there are any extra school year planners at his school. He decides to surprise me with his. This seems like it will be my best option. I will write down my most severe symptoms in all capital letters and my least pressing in small letters. I can also chart my medications, doctor's appointments, diet, menstrual cycle, and my yearly progress all at a month's glance. My ducks are all in a row. I am now completely ready to begin. Bring on the Guaifenesin.

## Starting the Guaifenesin

I have included the following monthly excerpts from my symptom journals. I can't stress enough how important keeping these journals becomes in validating and documenting your recovery. Enjoy!

## Thursday, August 14, 2003, Grand Haven, MI

This is my first official Guaifenesin Protocol journal entry. I am awake. It is 1:56 AM. I abruptly awoke to a distorted hissing sound that I didn't recognize. I took my first dose of Guaifenesin exactly thirteen hours ago. At first, this hissing noise shot through my ears, so I thought that it was something in the room. Now it won't stop. This symptom is new to me. I have never before experienced ringing in the ears. This is not at all the outcome that I had expected when I took my first dose of Guaifenesin earlier this evening before I went to bed. Could this be what Dr. St. Amand calls cycling, so soon? Is my body already reversing this illness by purging the calcium phosphate deposits? Am I cycling?

I am now fully awake. The Guaifenesin has heightened all of my senses. It's like someone has turned up the volume in my world. I am sure that I am cycling, which means that the calcium phosphate is leaving my body and the reversal process has begun. I am so excited. Yet I have to be honest: this is unpleasant. I am experiencing an extreme sensory overload. The once-dimly illuminated clock on my nightstand is suddenly blinding. Its reflection pierces through my eyes like a knife dipped into hot lava. As I close my eyes to soothe them, I hear my own breath. It is amplified like a fiery blowtorch. I desperately try to drown out all of the noises by placing cotton balls in each ear. No luck. All domestic noises are now foreign to me—the now constant droning of the dehumidifier in our basement (once only a faint buzz), the harsh roaring of our air conditioner outside our kitchen window (previously a hum), and the bellowing flush of our toilet (once a gentle swish).

Thirteen hours into my system, the Guaifenesin has become a speeding locomotive surging throughout my body with great force, destined to derail me, but I won't allow it. Unable to make it stop, I tell myself that the Guaifenesin is working and that this is a great occurrence.

All of my senses and all of my pain are heightened. In the darkness, I try to convince myself that good things are going to happen. This ringing in my ears is specific to me, and it confirms that the Guaifenesin is into my system and doing its job. In the darkness, I reassure myself that "Good things are going to come, Chantal, in time. The Guaifenesin is working."

## Sunday, August 17, 2003, Grand Haven, MI

I did not get dressed today. I have a horrible migraine headache that extends into the left side of my body, jaw, eye, face, neck, and shoulders. I am sore all over—from head to toe. The ringing in my ears won't stop. I am completely fogged. Once again, I am flat on my back in bed.

I am thankful that we have moved our bedroom downstairs into our office, since it adjoins a full bathroom. It is much easier for me not to have to climb the stairs. I am cycling so hard. The great news is that the Guaifenesin is working. It is doing its job. Rather than just having a fibromyalgia flare with more debris accumulating into my muscles, I am indeed experiencing what Dr. St. Amand refers to as cycling. I am getting the calcium phosphate OUT of my body. "Good things are going to come, Chantal!"

## Monday, August 18, 2003, Grand Haven, MI

My ankles, shins, and sciatic nerve are sore. My right thigh and buttock are incredibly painful. My headache is left-sided in the morning and then better in the evening. I am moody and angry and I want to be better this second! My thoughts are running rampant.

I am concerned about being *tolerably worse*. How will I know when I am tolerably worse? Will I become completely bedridden again? I hope not. I wonder what Dr. St. Amand meant when he stated that this protocol is not for the "faint at heart."

## September 2003

I am quickly finding out what Dr. St. Amand meant about this protocol not being for the "faint of heart." It takes diligence to keep the salicylates out of your life and a blind faith that the Guaifenesin is working.

But this is the key to the Guaifenesin Protocol. You actually have to make the Guai Protocol work for you, rather than just sitting back and letting it happen.

Some days the pain will be relentless, and that is when you need to reach deeper into your soul or call on a higher power for support. It's important to remember, when finding your correct dosage, that you should feel "tolerably worse" and yet still be able to function. You should not be "bedridden worse." Your cycles on Guaifenesin should never be worse than your worst flare-up before Guaifenesin. Be sure to be vigilant with your symptom journal. It's vital to keep it so you know what to look for to know when you are cycling. It's common to have too many symptoms all at once to know what is what. This is where the symptom journal comes in. You will eventually see a pattern. Aches and pains will shift. Fatigue levels will change. But, you won't realize any of this if you don't take the time to keep your journal. Your progress will be subtle, and you don't want to miss it. Take the time to record your symptoms. You will be grateful later.

Stay calm and give yourself pep talks. You can do this. Be patient and persistent. Don't allow yourself to listen to any negative self-doubts or those coming from others. Also follow the dosage schedule exactly as written. Don't up your dosage until the proper time. The idea is to have increased pain and symptoms but only to the point where they are *tolerably worse* and you can *still function*. You should not be bedridden at this point.

## October 2003

October is one of my absolute favorite months of the year. I love it when the leaves change color and the air cools. Halloween is also my most cherished holiday.

Unfortunately, right now, I am cycling so hard that I am too sick to get out of my pajamas and into my costume. I will remain inside the house, lights off, and drapes drawn until morning comes.

On the brighter side of things this month, I have been able to walk down my street almost every day. My appointments with Dr. Srutwa have also been going very well, and I can tell that acupuncture helps me very much energetically. I am completely off of Neurontin. I have been on it since September 2002. I gave it a good try. It did not help me at all. The first part of September, I was itchy and hot. Once again, I'm cycling like crazy, and this is a good thing.

I tried Botox for the first time for my migraines. Yikes! My newly tightened forehead, eagle eyebrows, and eyes don't suit me. I suppose it wouldn't be so bad if the Botox had actually helped my headaches, but it didn't. In fact, my migraines actually became worse as the week progressed. Go figure. Only me! I have to say that I am glad that I tried it. My neurologist informed me that sometimes relief is gained with the second set of injections. I will contemplate another round as the time nears. Thank you, God and the universe, for my health insurance that allowed me to try it.

## November 2003

I have had constant head, neck, and shoulder pain since I started the Guai in August 2003. My pain levels have been off the charts. In fact, I don't feel that I am *tolerably worse* and will talk to Dr. Srutwa about my dosage. Guaifenesin has gone over the counter, so the prescription Guai that I started with in August will soon be phased out. I am currently taking 1,800 mg of the Humibid prescription Guai.

Every day this month, I have been extremely light-sensitive, nauseated, and dizzy. I have been diligent with my walking routine and my tai chi stretches, because without them, I am just too stiff to function.

## December 2003

I am a bit concerned about how much energy I will have for Christmas shopping. With the added sensory overload, I am afraid that I just won't be able to handle it. My husband puts my worries to rest by giving me the go-ahead to shop online. Thank you, honey.

This month, cycling insomnia is at the forefront, even though I am diligent about keeping my blood sugar stable with an early morning slice of cheese, so it must be fibromyalgia and not my blood sugar. I have also had horrible bouts of extreme fatigue, constipation, hemorrhoids (which are not fibro related), plus a persistent yeast infection that didn't want to go away.

## January 2004

Happy New Year! Another month filled with extremes—extreme dry eyes, extreme fatigue, extreme nausea, extreme light sensitivity, extreme burning pain and stabbing pain, more muscle stiffness than usual, and pungent urine that I describe as the "phosphate smell." I am emotional and I feel as if I am going to die. It's not exactly a great way to start out the new year. But hope is here: I have the Guaifenesin Protocol.

New constant symptoms have emerged like pain in my arms, hands, and wrists. If I fall asleep with my hands in a fist position, then I have to pry them open in the morning. It's very strange.

I have my set appointments with Dr. Srutwa every Thursday morning, and he assures me that I am getting better despite my increase in symptoms. He is realizing, however, that I am not fitting the description of *tolerably worse* and that we are going to have to back down on my dosage of Guai. We can't figure out why my headaches are still so extreme. We have backed down on my dosage of Guai, and I am now taking 1,200 mg of Mucinex and have been for the past month. He also recommends that I try MSM powder for my hands *(www.swasnsonvitamins.com).* Although it is not part of the Guaifenesin Protocol, I think I will give it a try. It doesn't block the Guaifenesin and it should help my finger joints become less painful.

## February 2004

I began the MSM powder for my hands. My left pinky toe is burning. I must be cycling out this area. I broke that toe when I was in middle school. The Guai is doing its job.

I started Ambien 5 mg.

I had one visit to the ER this month for my bladder and vagina. I am experiencing cutting pain and pressure. My knees, feet, and shins are also hurting. My poor husband. One thing for sure is that life is never boring with me around our house. I also met with a new internist, a wonderful doctor who believes whole-heartedly in the spiritual side of wellness. Although he isn't familiar with the Guaifenesin Protocol and he is leery, he is open-minded and willing to learn. I am excited.

## March 2004

No pain in my hands for the first time in one and a half years! The MSM powder is working! Good visit with my internist. I sent my insurance company my reports from Dr. Srutwa's office in preparation for my disability hearing this month. I had been rejected my first time applying, and now it is my turn to appeal, so I have been requesting all of my records be sent to my disability representative.

## April 2004

Although I am cycling very hard this month, I have had a few better days and was able to scrape the wallpaper in our kitchen. I also had a week's worth of walks in, too. I am seeing the effects that gentle exercise really does help lower my pain levels. I am also clearly seeing the pattern in my symptom journal of fogginess, extreme fatigue, and dizziness the day after a diet cheat. Cheating on the HG diet and eating sugar also increases my pain levels.

I saw my internist again and Dr. Srutwa tried Biotape (*www.biotape.net*), even though it is not part of the Guaifeneisn Protocol, on my back and in between my shoulder blades. I mentioned that I would like to try the compounded MDR Guaifenesin sold by the Marina del Rey Pharmacy in California. I have been reading posts in the GauiGroup archives that mention that this Gaui is lactose- and dye-free, and I am thinking that the sudden surge in severity of my migraines might be due to the blue dye. Dr. Srutwa agrees to write me a prescription. Once it arrives in the mail, I will start over at 300 mg twice a day and evaluate my symptoms.

## May 2004

I believe that 300 mg twice a day of the MDR Guai is my cycling dose. I feel *tolerably worse.* My migraines and light sensitivity are still my most challenging fibromyalgia symptoms. They make walking outdoors un-enjoyable most days, although, I did walk almost everyday this month and I am proud of myself.

## June 2004

I received great news today through the mail that I won my disability hearing. I am so relieved. Josh and I are celebrating—ironically—with chocolate chip cookies. I know: I know I will pay for this tomorrow in the form of increased IBS symptoms, fatigue, anxiety, problems with memory and concentration, pain, and possibly a horrible migraine. This has been a tough month for me, with tons of pain and extreme fatigue. I blocked deliberately for one week by using a para-cleanse in the hopes of getting rid of my light sensitivity. The doctors still can't say for sure whether my light sensitivity is caused by the fibromyalgia or something else. I am constantly hoping that something will alleviate it.

## July 2004

More vaginal burning, nausea, dizziness, throbbing hands, and pain from head to toe. My internist decides to stop my extended-release Metformin that I have been taking for the past six years for polycystic ovarian syndrome (not related to my fibromyalgia). I am to note any change in headaches once stopped.

## August 2004

Great month! We held our first official fibromyalgia/Guaifenesin Protocol support group meeting this month. It was a success. We had six members in attendance. We will continue to hold them every third Saturday at 10 AM, with a break for the winter holiday.

## Thursday, August 12, 2004, Grand Haven, MI

Today is my thirty-fifth birthday. In two days, I will be celebrating my first year on Guaifenesin. June marked my first year on the hypoglycemic diet. I have lost forty pounds, and my cholesterol numbers and blood tests are all normal.

Although I still have a headache every day, I notice that the severity of it has decreased considerably. I am sure that I was sensitive to the blue dye. The acupuncture has really helped me energetically. I did have a bite of cake and ice cream today, and I am paying for it in the form of increased head pain, anxiety, day sweats, and pounding heart. I can predict what tomorrow will bring. Yes, my irritable bowel syndrome will be acting up in the form of explosive gas. That is when I will ask myself, "Was it really worth it?" But since it still is my birthday, I won't dwell on that now. I will just enjoy my progress from this past year.

## September 2004

I began physical therapy. I think that this is really going to help my sciatica. My goal is to be able to walk upright without hunching over due to pain in my right sacroiliac joint. I like my trainer. He doesn't know exactly what to make of me, though. I am his first patient with fibromyalgia and his only patient who has ever presented with extreme photophobia. He is my age, patient, and kind, and gives me a very reassuring grin each time I arrive in his office wearing my sunglasses and hat.

My bladder is burning and out of control. I feel like I have a bladder infection, but I also realize that my eyes are burning. This must be more intense cycling. I have a prescription for Pyridium to take for bladder emergencies. I take one and my symptoms lessen. I decide to stop the Guai for one day to see how I feel. I know that my body might be slammed when I restart, but I need to see how I feel without it in my system.

My bladder symptoms are better today without the Guai. This confirms that it was cycling. I will mentally brace myself and restart it tomorrow.

## October 2004

I started walking again on October 1. I try to do ten to twenty minutes each day, outside. Dr. Srutwa says that it is vital to start restoring my energy supply. I also do his tai chi exercises daily. It hurts to move, but I am doing it. I also started the new dye-free lactose-free Marina Del Rey Pharmacy Guai today. Although I have had upper back pain, heartburn, and burning eyes all this week, I am thrilled to be getting off some of these prescription drugs.

In my detailed symptom journal, I am noticing that if I have a diet cheat, I am foggy the next day. It does not matter how small the cheat or what protein combos I try to add to it, such as a bite of cheese or meat, after I eat something sweet. *My body knows.*

## November 2004

What a month! I had a completely unnerving gynecological exam on the tenth of November. I nearly left the office rattled and in tears.

This doctor told me that my husband should absolutely have a vasectomy and that we should not have any kids because of my fibromyalgia. She told me that if I am sick now with it, pregnancy will only make my condition worse and that there is no way that I can ever have my own children. I must give up that hope. Needless to say, I fired her.

November has been filled with physical therapy appointments, reflexology, acupuncture, soft-tissue manipulation, trigger-point injections, increased fatigue, major TMJ pain, and increased light sensitivity. My internist has decided to taper me off of the Toprol for my blood pressure and start me on Verapimil instead. We are hoping that this will help me with my light sensitivity as one of the known side effects of Toprol is light sensitivity.

## December 2004

My bladder has been horrible. I am cycling like crazy. Pyridium to the rescue! I am continuing with my weekly physical therapy, acupuncture, soft-tissue manipulation, myofascial pain release, and reflexology. Overall, I am noticing slight improvements in my arms, hands, and wrists.

## January 2005

Happy New Year 2005! This month my main symptoms are bladder, headache, light sensitivity, insomnia, nausea, and dizziness. I also have a follow up appointment with my internist. I am itchy from head to toe, and Claudia, author and moderator of the GuaiGroup, has reassured me that this is due to cycling. I am purging the calcium phosphate out of my body, and this is a very good thing. I am to take more lukewarm showers and baths, be patient, and in time this will go.

I am starting to see more patterns in my symptom journal, and although I still feel like a Mack truck has hit me daily, I am getting better. Last month, I was hit with apathy and didn't feel like logging many of my symptoms. The constant ringing in my ears lets me know that the Guai is still working.

## February 2005

This month has been all about my bladder and cycling. I met with my internist to have my urine tested to rule out a bladder infection. It is not a bladder infection. I have increased my water intake and have tried Pyridium.

My headaches are consistent and it makes sense that they will be the last symptom for me to cycle out, since I have had them since I was five or six years old. We cycle out our most recent symptoms first.

## March 2005

This month I have been on an emotional rollercoaster. I must be cycling my emotions. It sounds strange, but yes, we do cycle the calcium phosphate deposits in the brain and with that comes the emotional rollercoaster. I am weepy. Everything seems to be hitting me all at once. We have our house up for sale, and I have to face the fact that next month, I will have to officially resign from my job. My MESSA health insurance through work will stop at the end of this month. But I am fortunate to still have health insurance through my husband's job. He is also a teacher and teaches in Grand Rapids, Michigan, about an hour away by car. He has been commuting since we got married in July 2001, but has decided that it will be more practical and financially better for us if we move to the city where he works. Josh hopes to find a house by June, so we can be all moved in by August when the new school year begins. He doesn't want to continue his commute especially with the price of gas at $2.00 a gallon.

I met with my internist again to talk about my progress and learn some new meditative techniques. I feel that any therapy that I can utilize will help in my overall wellbeing and I am willing to try almost anything to get well as long as it doesn't block the Guaifenesin.

Dr. Srutwa has moved and expanded his office to include a wide range of other medical professionals. I have decided to give homeopathic medicine a try, since it won't block the Guai. I will do almost anything to try to rid myself of my light sensitivity. I also began seeing a chiropractor who uses an activator machine on me.

Little by little, I have been packing up our house. We are hoping to put it on the market by May. I really don't want to move, but my three-year time limit to keep my job as a high school teacher will expire in April. I am not yet well enough to go back to work. I am still suffering on a daily basis from extreme fatigue, insomnia, light sensitivity, noise sensitivity, migraine headaches, and bladder symptoms. I will miss my local doctors and support system here.

## April 2005

I am cycling my emotions. I am angry and feel stressed. I also have tons of heartburn and vertigo. Josh took me to visit my adopted Grandpa Bob, who is eighty-eight years young. Ironically, he is the one who drove me to my disability hearing last year.

## May 2005

I celebrated this month with bronchitis, swollen feet, itchy toes, TMJ, bladder issues, sinus pressure, right hip pain, nausea, and a sore neck, head, and shoulders. I continued with my physical therapy and appointments with Dr. Srutwa. I called around getting estimates for our mortgage loan, and for the first time in almost three years, my headache vanished for one day!

## June 2005

My sister Michelle is getting married in August, and I am in her wedding. I am hoping that I will see some improvement in the next two months. I don't know how I am going to wear heels with my feet cycling as hard as they have been. I am also heat intolerant, so I don't know how I am going to function in the small mountain church without air conditioning. Her bridal shower was this month, and I fared pretty well. Although I am on the strict hypoglycemic diet, my headaches have still been relentless. Dr. Srutwa mapped some lumps at the base of my skull that he thinks are partially responsible for my head pain. I am hoping that I will clear this area soon.

Josh and I found a house in Grand Rapids, and we put an offer in on it. We had it inspected, and it did not pass inspection. So we are going to have our second choice inspected this week.

We made an offer on house number two and it was accepted. We take possession immediately at close, and we are closing in July. We had our first open house with our Grand Haven house and no bites.

## July 2005

We closed on our new house and I made arrangements to have a radon fan installed, laminate floorings installed, and the electrical updated with a new box and three prong sockets. Everything is happening so quickly. I am feeling emotional and worried that my health progress will be stalled if I move away from my doctors and support system.

## August 2005

I am definitely doing more this month. Little by little, I am getting better. I painted and pulled staples at the new house. I rode while Josh drove, over two thousand miles round trip to our cottage in Mont-Tremblant, Quebec, Canada, to participate in my youngest sister's wedding, as a matron of honor. Yes, I survived the rehearsal dinner, the beauty shop, fancy heels, her ceremony, and the reception clean-up with sunglasses on. My sister got married at 11 AM. The day was a scorching-hot, mid-August day, without air conditioning inside the tiny mountain chapel, but the wedding was ever so beautiful. As soon as I made my way to the reception hall, my fancy heels were off. It was a fourteen-hour production and something that I would not have made it through even one year ago.

But hooray for me, and thank God and the universe for the Guaifenesin Protocol!

## September 2005

E.R.

Bladder, bladder, bladder and more bladder issues without infection. Welcome to the world of interstitial cystitis, Chantal, combined with cycling the Guai! I stopped the Guai to give my bladder a break, although this isn't the best thing to do, because the restarting of the Guai can really slam you. But after two straight weeks of bladder nonsense and Pyridium for pain, I've had enough, and I will take my chances with the restart.

## October 2005

October is my most favorite month of the year. I love to watch the leaves change color and make their final descent. This year is the first in the past seven that I will be living close enough to my mom's house to be able to partake in her Halloween night festivities. I can't wait to celebrate with my family. We always have a large birthday party for my mom, whose birthday is the thirtieth of October. Halloween is a grand event for us, full of creativity, warmth, and family fun. We all dress up to pass out candy and decorate her front yard with lights that create a path with lawn chairs (where we sit to pass out the candy) which lead up to her front porch. Even Bob, my adopted grandfather, who is in his eighties, dresses up and passes out candy with us. The trick-or-treaters love this.

We had a great night celebrating. I did eat a couple of mini chocolates and will be paying for it tomorrow with increased bodily pain and headache.

In fact, I've had a couple diet cheats this month and a bad sinus/migraine when I restarted the Guai after stopping it for bladder issues. (I don't recommend stopping the Guai.) Acupuncture, acupuncture, and more acupuncture does this fibromyalgic body good and I still go weekly.

## November 2005

One diet cheat with donuts, and for the following four days, I felt like death warmed over. Those donuts were *so* not worth it! Otherwise, it was a good month with some irritable (IBS) issues that truly correspond to the diet donut cheats!

## December 2005

This was a crazily busy month. New doctors: OB-GYN and a new internist. I like these two new doctors. The new internist is super smart, logical, and open-minded. I haven't approached him with my fibro yet, but will in time. This new OB-GYN told me that if I want to have a baby, I could absolutely have one. She has had patients with fibromyalgia who have actually felt *better* while pregnant. I just need to do it before I am forty years old. She is familiar with fibro, but not the Guaifenesin Protocol. I have appointments with Dr. Srutwa and another in-town acupuncturist. Tons of lower back pain and upper right shoulder blade area pain cycling. Head, neck, and shoulders hurt. I have extreme fatigue for a few days, but the acupuncture really helps me on an energetic level.

## January 2006

I had tons of issues this month. I am cycling like *crazy!* Insomnia is my chief complaint, followed by nausea, upper back tightness, bladder, IBS, and migraine with aura.

## February 2006

More episodes of migraine with aura, and I am starting to see a correlation with my blood sugar dipping too low and that left-sided weak feeling and numbness in the face. Interesting. Extreme fatigue, heartburn, head, neck, shoulders, neurological numbness, and right hip pain. Cycling?

## March 2006

Indoor house painting this month, filled with bladder issues once again. Arms, hands, wrists are killing me and so stiff—due to the painting. This month is filled with headaches, nausea, and acupuncture. We are still trying to sell our old house and have switched Realtors.

## April 2006

We got a dog, Kaari, a medium-sized black dog, a cocker spaniel/lab mix! I needed something to mother. Josh named him after a Viking dude. I am still adjusting to having a dog in the house, since I've never had one before. I need to register us for obedience classes. Pain levels have improved, and not too many symptoms to report this month. Thank you, Guaifenesin Protocol!

## May 2006

A few diet cheats and related consequences of IBS, night sweats, and heart palpitations. So not worth the cheat!

## June 2006

This is a sad month. My father-in-law, Neil Sanders, passed away after a long and painful battle with multiple myeloma cancer. I still can't believe he is gone. What a huge loss.

# Part 5

## Re-inventing Self

# Chapter 5: The Fifth Step: Stepping Out of the Fibromyalgia Story

"Be the change you wish to see in the world."
—Mahatama Gandhi

"Do not wait; the time will never be just right. Start where you stand and work with whatever tools you have at your command and better tools will be found as you go along."
—George Herbert

## Practicing Personal Empowerment

"Where did *you* start? How did *you* put your life back together while following the Guaifenesin Treatment Protocol? What did *you* do?" As the leader of a Fibromyalgia/Guaifenesin Protocol support group here in Michigan, I have been asked these same three questions many times over the years.

Overwhelmed, frustrated, fatigued, forlorn, hesitant, and cautious, these individuals look to me for pointers on where to begin. Their very natural fear of the unknown, combined with fibro-fogged brains and a lack of self-confidence, holds them back from initially beginning the protocol.

They tell me that they are afraid that the cycling stage (purging of the calcium phosphates from their bodies), once taking the Guaifenesin, will be too intense for them to handle. If they are hypoglycemic, they have doubts about changing their diets, lack the energy to cook, and simply don't believe that they can do it. They are worried that their families won't understand their blood sugar problems and support their new way of eating. They are overwhelmed, isolated, desperate, and drained.

I always reassure them that their concerns are completely normal and that I once held them too, but I didn't let my fear hold me back. I knew that I would only get worse over time. After all, there is currently no cure for fibromyalgia. It's not going away, and prescription medications in many cases, only provide a temporary solution. But it can be reversed with the Guaifenesin, and they can do it themselves. I share with them that many people—thousands, to be exact—have gotten their lives back. Dr. St. Amand has made fibromyalgia recovery his life's mission, and he is currently in his third year of a three-year research study to isolate the genes in fibromyalgia and to develop a diagnostic blood test. I knew six years ago when I began the protocol that I had nothing to lose by trying the Guaifenesin and only my life to gain. So I went for it. And am I glad that I did!

At first it wasn't easy, but I completely believe that we ultimately attract what we put out into the universe by our thoughts and that we can use them to re-invent ourselves, to reclaim our personal value, and to create our own perfect health.

For me, starting the Guaifenesin Protocol began with the following two mantras: "Be the change that you wish to see in the world" by Mahatama Gandhi and "Do not wait; the time will never be just right. Start where you stand and work with whatever tools you have at your command and better tools will be found as you go along," by George Herbert. Together these two quotes gave me the strength that I needed to begin the Guaifenesin Protocol.

So I decided to become the change that I wished to see, and I did not wait to start. In fact, I started nine months before I had even received my official diagnosis of fibromyalgia. I started exactly where I was standing, or in my case, I started exactly where I was lying down, alone and in the dark, on that futon mattress on our living room floor.

It wasn't easy. In the beginning, for the first three months, every morning after my husband left for work, I grieved and sobbed. I cried out loud while trying to make sense of this mysterious illness. My cats were my only companions. They didn't understand my fits of rage and my howling, but they faithfully remained by my side. I was so angry and frustrated, I wanted to scream, "Why me? How did I get here? What did I do to deserve this?" But instead, I sat in silence. Some days the quiet was deafening and seemed to make my pain worse. I was at the nadir of my existence, about to give up, when something remarkable happened.

I decided to step back, take a deep breath, and be in the present moment with my anger. I surrendered my need to be in control. I stopped battling with the invisible. Instead of fighting my health situation, I accepted it as *right now.* I let go of the resistance. I changed my perspective. I put my hope out there. I took a giant leap of faith. I silenced all of the "should haves" and the "could haves" in my brain. I did not give up. No, instead I decided that I would now use my anger and my frustration as tools to help me become well again. It sounds strange, but I used my anger to get well.

Instead of my anger being my enemy, I made it my friend. Like a jet pack strapped to my back, I allowed myself to release my anger and turn it into engine fuel to propel myself up, forward, and out. I made peace with the unknown, this mysterious illness. I stopped struggling and I accepted myself—"I am that I am."

I knew that I wouldn't be sick forever, that this wouldn't last forever. This was just a bump right now in my road called life. I never looked back. I never got stuck on self-pity. Sure, I would have my moments of despair. But hope was out there for me somewhere, and I would find it. Deep down, I knew that I held the power inside of myself to become well again.

I thought of Dorothy in *The Wizard of OZ* and her astonishment when she realized that she was wearing the magic ruby slippers and that she had always possessed the power to tap them together to go home. She had always had this force inside of her; she just didn't realize it. I learned from her.

I knew that I held this type of positive energy inside of me in the form of my thoughts and my perspective. How I viewed my situation and the course that I decided to take with it was my choice. My thoughts were within my management. I could either allow myself to become the victim and crawl into a dark hole, engulfed with apprehension and helplessness, or I could put on my pair of marvelous ruby-red slippers and believe, believe that I could get well.

I chose the glistening ruby slippers. No longer able to care for myself, to read, or to write, I decided rather than become depressed, I would just shift my perspective. Let go of the old me. You may be wondering how I did that. How could I just let go of the old me?

At first, this was no simple task. It came slowly, minute by minute, some days second by second. I no longer allowed my emotions to deplete me of the little remaining energy that I had left. Instead, I decided to be in the present moment and one with my pain and fatigue. And I accepted them. Now this does not mean that I gave up or that the pain or the fatigue went away. On the contrary, I made the conscious decision to get well, to change, and to become unstuck.

Once officially diagnosed with fibromyalgia, I knew that I had nothing to lose by trying the Guaifenesin Protocol, and that my feelings were the most prominent tools at my command. They were my thoughts, and I knew that I could change them. I could stop the self-blame of "How did I get here?" I could stop the incessant mind chatter and feelings of guilt about not being able to contribute to the family financially anymore. I could stop beating myself up for being a failure. And I could remember that I was lucky and show my gratitude. I was still alive. I had a loving husband, a young stepson who adored me, and three cats that never left my side. I could do this. I could try this new treatment and make it successful.

Take the time you need to mourn what you have lost, but don't get stuck in it. Don't let it consume you. The more you focus on how sick you are, the sicker you could very possibly become. Change your focus. Shift your thoughts. Become the change that you wish to see. Empower yourself. Use whatever tools you have at your command. Focus on the fact that you are doing the Guaifenesin Treatment Protocol and that you are making it work. Have faith in yourself. Be proud. Keep your eyes focused on the goal: perfect health. Stand tall. Let patience become your most cherished virtue.

## Meeting Support

At my four-month marker of being on the Guaifenesin Protocol, I was finally beginning to be able to read and to write again (thanks to the hypoglycemic diet, Ambien, and Flexeril), and better tools were coming along into my life, despite the fact that I still felt so gravely ill.

This is when I met Almeda, my local doctor's one and only other fibromyalgia patient. After months of daily phone conversations, there we were, finally standing face to face in his office. We had inadvertently scheduled our appointments back to back that day, and we were both thrilled to finally meet!

Though she was forty years my senior and six months ahead of me on the Guaifenesin Protocol, we instantly became good friends. We both had hit rock bottom with our fibromyalgia/chronic fatigue syndrome and were more than ready to begin something new. We were Dr. Srutwa's first and only fibromyalgia patients to try the Guaifenesin.

We both dove into the Guaifenesin Protocol, and because we both had hypoglycemia, we both clung on to the diet as if it was a life preserver thrown overboard to us. (In fact, it was!)

We called each other daily, sometimes more than once. Our conversations always lasted an hour and revolved around creating new hypoglycemic diet-friendly recipes and trying them out on each other. We each kept a symptom journal and compared notes. With her help, I further empowered myself. I got out of my box. I stepped out of my fibromyalgia story. Thank you, Almeda.

Because talking on the phone was one of the only activities that each of us could do, because we were both so sick, together with our doctor, the three of us decided to start a Fibromyalgia/Guaifenesin Protocol support group for his patients, which consisted only of the two of us and then one other man that first year. We knew that we could lend fibromyalgia support via the telephone. And that is exactly what we both did.

That first year, we tested the "Guaifenesin Protocol waters" first by supporting each other, finding our correct dosages, creating new, yummy HG-friendly recipes, keeping our symptom journals, and comparing notes. We gained confidence in the protocol and were becoming well enough that we knew we needed to expand.

Word was quickly spreading in our small lakeshore town that there was a local medical doctor who believed in fibromyalgia/chronic fatigue syndrome. In fact, Dr. Srutwa was combining his expertise of soft-tissue manipulation and acupuncture to treat his patients, while they gradually reversed their fibromyalgia by following the protocol. Wholeheartedly, Dr. Strutwa believed in Dr. St. Amand's work, but most importantly, he believed in us. So we expanded our telephone support group to online, and then eventually we began holding monthly Fibromyalgia/Guaifenesin Protocol meetings at his office. It is very important to find support during your reversal process. To be in the company of like minds is essential during your recovery, whether it is via an online support group or over the telephone. No one understands fibromyalgia like those who have it.

Needless to say, I was at the helm again and back to "teaching," all volunteer, in a completely different way and loving it. I was happy and grateful. My progress was slow and steady. This protocol really did work, as long as I worked it.

I was determined, and I vowed to myself that one day, although I wasn't certain about the exact time frames, one day I was going to get well enough—well enough to travel to California and personally meet and thank the genius behind this Guaifenesin Treatment Protocol and well enough to have my own child.

## Learning to Ask for Help

I have always considered myself a very independent woman, and asking for help was something that I despised ever doing. I was forever the caregiver in my family while growing up, happily meeting the needs of others and chauffeuring everyone else around. But then fibromyalgia/ chronic fatigue syndrome entered my world and stripped me of all that.

In the fall of 2003, sick with debilitating migraines, bodily pain, and fatigue, thirteen months had passed and I had not driven myself anywhere fun. In fact, I was bedridden, housebound, and desperately needed a change.

Still somewhat in denial of the severity of my fibro-fogged brain and newly diagnosed illness, I foolishly ventured out on my own. My goal for the day was to go to our local Meijer grocery store and pick up a few items. Meijer stores are equivalent in size to Super Wal-Marts or Kmarts. They are expansive.

I remember pulling into the parking lot and then walking into the store. As soon as I entered the store, I was instantly blown away by sensory overload. I felt my face flush and my legs become limp like cooked spaghetti. Overwhelmed, my mind blanked, and I had no idea how I had gotten there or how I was going to be able to get myself home. Instinct told me to turn around and head straight for the parking lot. I was in trouble.

In the parking lot, I couldn't find my car. This was in the days before I had a panic button on my key chain. I felt shaky. I was dizzy and couldn't concentrate. My body was beginning to pour with sweat. My head was pounding even more, and I felt as if I was going to pass out. So much for venturing out on my own! Now what was I going to do?

My husband worked an hour away by car, and there was no way that he could help me now. The only friends I had in town were teachers, and they were all working. I was embarrassed. I didn't know what to do. Should I go back into the store and ask the greeter for help? Explain to him that I get very bad migraines and have fibromyalgia and I sometimes become disorientated and forget how to do things?

*Try to think, Chantal, think. Take a deep breath. What am I going to do? Where did I park that car?* I was desperate. I had never done this sort of thing before; I had never gone to a destination and then completely forgotten where I was or how I was going to get home. This was new to me. So I decided to start calling out for help in my mind. Yes, I started calling, "God, I need help. I need an angel right now! I need an angel right now!" That is when I heard it—I heard someone call my name. In a very chipper and happy voice, I heard, "Hi, Chantal!"

I turned to see who was speaking to me in such a sweet tone. It was Kim, the daughter of my former kindergarten teacher. I had not seen her for twelve years or so, and I had actually forgotten that she lived in the Tri-Cities area. I couldn't believe my luck. Now, how do I tell someone that I haven't seen for twelve years that I am sick and I can't find my car, that I need help, and I don't think that I will be able to drive my car home? Ugh …

Fortunately, I didn't have to say a word. She could tell by my expression and my body language that something was gravely wrong. She later told me that I looked as if I was in severe pain. She offered to give me a ride home. I told her that that would be great, but that I needed to find my car first. It was somewhere in the parking lot. By the time we found it, I was calm enough to drive myself home. She followed me, just in case.

A couple weeks later, I got up the courage to ask Kim if I could go with her to the store when she did her weekly shopping. Every Monday for the next three years, she became my shopping buddy. She would pick me up, and we would go shopping together. This became my only outing and social contact for the week. Prior to my fibromyalgia "crash," I never would have considered asking for help in this way. Don't be afraid to ask for help. Asking for help is not a sign of failure or weakness. I needed her support and friendship. I could not have done it without her. Thank you, Kim.

## Finding Unconditional Support

One Saturday afternoon, after my eight-year-old stepson's football practice, he arrived home all smiles. This was an odd reaction from him, since he did not enjoy football practice, and I immediately knew something was brewing.

That is when he proudly displayed in his hands the ugliest, tiny gray and calico-striped furball I had ever seen. (And I love cats and kittens!) She was obviously the runt of the litter, scruffy and very flea-infested.

"Who's this?" I asked.

"Lily," Nikolaus replied as he proceeded to tell me that he and Dad had gone to the Humane Society after his game. They were just going "to look" at the animals, but it was closed for a special dog adoption event. As luck would have it, a lady was dropping off this kitten at the exact same time that they were driving into the parking lot. When she realized that the shelter was closed, she asked Nikolaus if he wanted the kitten. She explained that her son was allergic and they couldn't keep her. She gave them a free bag of kitten chow and Dad said yes.

Our house soon became a three-cat house, and I was not ready for this type of a surprise. Taking care of myself these days was hard enough. Although I love cats, I did not need another mouth to feed. I did not need the responsibility of another pet. Soon my attitude changed.

Let me tell you about Lily. Her joy of life is infectious. When she purrs all of her tiny three-pound body vibrates like a cell phone tucked in a pocket. She loves to nestle on my chest and nuzzle under my chin whenever I am lying down, and these days, it is often. Her lack of depth perception and bursts of sudden energy make her kittenish bounds something out of a cartoon. When startled she stands back arched, fur erect, and leaps straight up into the air, and then lands all four legs sprawled midair. She is quite amusing and provides the comic relief that my body craves.

One day, she decided to use my housecoat as a climbing post while I was wearing it. You can only imagine my split-second horror as I stood motionless in our living room one morning, as I watched what appeared to be a tiny gray streak at the opposite end of the house, charging toward me. Yes, in one fell swoop, Lily managed to climb, claws fully deployed, all the way up my fleece robe and onto my shoulder. Luckily, the robe was thick.

Needless to say, I am enchanted. And although I still have extreme pain and fatigue, I am happy again with this newfound support. I am no longer alone. I talk to her all day long, and she responds with a few quick meows as if she knows what I am saying.

The older cats find her annoying and want nothing to do with her. I find her adorable and can't get enough of her. She's bringing the joy back into my heart and is creating a wonderful distraction for me, away from my daily pain and fatigue.

If at all possible, I highly recommend adopting a pet from your local shelter or borrowing one from a neighbor. They will do wonders for your mental health and well-being, love you just the way you are, and take your focus off of yourself.

## Creating to be Pain-free

Nine months after beginning the Guaifenesin Protocol, in my pursuit of health and answers, I met another fantastic doctor who believed in the spiritual side of wellness. He introduced me to Bruce Lipton, PhD, and his book, *The Biology of Belief.* Lipton believed that disease was five percent genetic and seventy percent "dis-ease." (Lipton 2005, pp.123-144). He taught me that, "While we can't control our genetics, we can control our thoughts."

Instead of asking me if I was *depressed,* like all of the other doctors had done this past year, he asked me if I was *angry.*

My first response was, "No." Since I had accepted my situation and felt hopeful that I would reverse my fibromyalgia and become well again, I was no longer angry that I was sick.

That is not what he meant. What he wanted to know was, *did I have any previous anger that I was holding on to?*

*Duh, doesn't everyone? Isn't this normal?* I thought to myself.

I felt my stomach drop. I felt my face flush with panic. I had anger bottled up inside me, sure, years and years of it. But I never thought that these things were stunting my recovery, as I didn't think about these people or situations on a daily basis.

He explained to me his belief that depression and anger are cousins and that some forms of depression are just forms of anger that have never been expressed or released.

I had homework to do. He gave me my assignment. I was to get a journal and write, even if my struggles with fibro-fog made that difficult. I was to change my perspective and forgive these people. He said I could take the next few months if I needed to, but it had to be done. I had to let go of the hurt and the pain. I had to learn to forgive in order to move forward.

I was to begin by writing the person's name and the incident, however unpleasant it was. Just jot down the name and the experience, as many as I could recall. Leave some space in between each entry. Take my time. I could fill the whole journal if necessary.

First I had to revisit every incident and write it only from *my point of view.* Next I had to state why I thought the other person had acted the way he or she did from *his or her point of view.* How did it make me feel? What did I think of them for it? And finally and most importantly of all, *what had I learned from the experience and how has it changed me for the better?*

I spent hours on this one. It was homework that flowed. Yes, I was full of anger. And I was more than ready to rid myself of it.

I brought my journal to my next appointment. My doctor was pleased with it, and I felt lighter and proud for the first time in months. He was happy to see that I was learning to let go of anger and the "dis-ease," learning to forgive, and developing my spiritual side.

He had another homework assignment for me, but first he wanted to review my blood work and to talk more about the Guaifenesin Protocol. I had been following the Guaifenesin Protocol and the hypoglycemic diet for nine months now, and my blood tests were becoming closer to normal.

In the course of a year, I watched my triglycerides fall from 458 to 222 and then to 140. I lost forty pounds. I felt lighter, both physically and emotionally, despite the daily horrendous pain and fatigue. I knew that I was making gradual but steady progress and that someday my story would help to inspire others.

My next homework assignment from this doctor was to get back in touch with my creative side. Buy some crayons; just scribble out my emotions on a sketch pad; close my eyes and draw. I was not to worry about the composition. Choose the colors that match my emotions in this moment, in the now, and scribble. Place no judgments on myself or on what I have created. The main goal here is to be in the now, to create and to do.

"You are now to put all that you have learned into practice. I want you to do, do, do! Do something that you love to do every day!"

I bought a sketchbook for myself, my first one in about ten years. I felt a giddy excitement build as I walked down the art supply aisle. I was relieved to see that sketchbooks hadn't changed at all. *Ah, finally something familiar.*

I also purchased Mark Kistler's basic drawing book online and practiced making pencil shapes in it. Yes, you read that right—basic shapes and scribbles. Eventually I expanded my art tools to include colored pencils.

At first it was disheartening for me to believe that I was now retraining myself how to scribble. How could this be? Where had the person gone, that artist who used to sell her artwork, who was one class short of a major in art from Western Michigan University?

She was now learning how to scribble again. Yes, me, scribble!

So I decided to re-evaluate and change my thoughts and expectations of myself once again. I was here to let go of my fears and to stop judging myself. Yes, it was finally time for me to start being kind to myself and to love myself, just as Dr. Srutwa, my local doctor, had recommended. It was time for me to learn to cut myself some slack and love myself.

Eventually, I did get back into my artwork, and now, almost seven years later, I am creating motivational, affirmational cards and signs for fun, using vibrant acrylic washes. I like this new creative me.

This assignment was not as easy as it sounds. It did not flow like the fibromyalgia forgiveness journal. In fact, at first I had to force myself to close my eyes and draw. I had to restart several times. But in time I learned. I learned to let go of my ego. Letting go of my ego is still a work in progress because it filters into all areas of my life. I am still a work in progress, and that is okay. The creativity blockage that I developed happened over time. I ignored my spirit. I pushed myself through college. Then I pushed myself through graduate school. I pushed myself through student teaching. I pushed myself through everything, and in the process of the pushing, I lost myself. My creativity was zero. That little voice inside me that said "You are worth it" was dead.

## Doing Something You Love Every Day

Doing something you love every day is a great way to create a pain-free distraction. Find ways in your life to do something that you love every day. No matter what stage of this illness you are in, you always have the power to invent ways to be creative.

Early on in my illness, I took out one of my old notebooks for teaching, and rather than wallowing in the fact that I could no longer use it for teaching, I decorated it to make an inspiration/vision board. It took me a week to decorate the cover. From travel magazines that were still being sent to our house, I embellished it with scenes of faraway places that I dreamt of one day visiting, even though I could no longer travel. I didn't let this get me down. Instead, I filled the cover with inspirational words. I found my favorite photo of Nueschwanstein Castle in Germany (the same castle Walt Disney used for his castle design) and hung it on my fridge. I focused on my goal that once well I would go on a castle tour of Europe with my husband. Yes, these tours do exist, and you can even stay overnight in the castles!

I thought of other ways that I could pull myself out of my isolation and channel my frustration to change my thoughts and my perspective. I dug out the hand-held, voice- activated tape recorder that I had gotten to take with me to Mayo Clinic to record my appointments. Although I never used it for that purpose, I now found a new use for it.

Since I was desperately in need of a friend during the day while I was home alone, I decided to dictate my story to myself to try to make sense out of it. So I placed it on my bathroom countertop while I bathed. This seemed to be the only time my mind was clear enough to get my thoughts on tape. Although my mysterious illness had taken so much from me, I was determined I wasn't going to let it win. I would be the victor, not the victim, and I would let it teach me.

I focused on the few activities that I was still able to do, like taking a bath, talking on the phone, snuggling up with my cats, and pulling the comforter up over my bed every day.

Yes, in those initial fibromyalgia crash days of reverting back into infancy, I gave myself permission to enroll in kindergarten again—home alone in the dark on the futon mattress on the floor. I meditated; I sat in silence; I prayed. I learned to enjoy the stillness. I believed that I would find my answers and get my diagnosis eventually, and rather than beat myself up and focus on loss or allow myself to become depressed, I concentrated on the thought of learning something new through my foggy brain, and this was both terrifying and exciting!

Eventually I got my official diagnosis of fibromyalgia, and I was introduced to the Guaifenesin Protocol. In the meantime, however, I taught myself to sew with a sewing machine, although I had to remind my foggy brain each time I used it how to thread the needle and to rethread the bobbin. I enjoyed making pillows and bags, and I found my days no longer dragged quite as much.

I also took up crocheting with a giant hook. My grandma had taught me this as a child, and it must have been stuck in my long-term memory, as it was an activity that I actually could remember how to do. The only difference now was the size of the hook. It was jumbo sized, and I needed it that way.

This massive hook was big enough that I could use it with my arthritic-like fibromyalgic hands, which would by morning be so stiff that I would have to literally pry them open if I had fallen asleep with them in a fist-like position. This larger hook worked out well, and I was pleased with my projects: a cotton blanket for my cats and a rug for our laundry room made out of recycled plastic shopping bags. Although I was pleased with my projects, I continued to remind myself that this illness was just a bump in my road of life. I would learn to do simple things and to draw again. In time, I would eventually get my life back, and I would one day meet Dr. St. Amand and Claudia Craig Marek.

But I quickly found out that getting my life back wasn't just about learning how to express my creativity again while doing the Guaifenesin Protocol. It was also more than keeping the symptom journal, eliminating salicylates from my life, and being mapped. Re-inventing myself also meant that I had to begin to meet the challenge of creating some normalcy in my life. This meant that I needed to start from scratch to relearn how to do simple things to feel successful. Yes, I needed to set a daily routine, with the same start and end times each day, with a daily goal or two to accomplish.

## Discovering the Joy of Movement

Finding my specific "joy of movement" has been one of my most vital steps in reversing my fibromyalgia/chronic fatigue syndrome and returning to perfect health. I discovered my specific style at my five-year marker. I seriously urge you to find time to stretch and to move today, no matter what your pain or fatigue levels. Hindsight has taught me that I should not have waited until my fifth year on the protocol, because gentle exercise like walking produces energy in our fibromyalgic bodies. Create a joy of movement that works for you. Here is one of my posts to the GuaiGroup:

> Hello Fellow Guaiers,
>
> I feel fantastic—exercise! I've caught myself several times now within the past few months uttering those words and I wanted to share, as I can't believe my own transformation.
>
> I had read many posts in the past years while on the Guaifenesin Protocol about exercise and how beneficial it is for us, but every time that I attempted it, my elliptical machine, my exercise bike, videos etc…I failed and it—exercise—left me in pain for days.
>
> In my fibromyalgic world, taking a shower, getting dressed, and blow-drying my hair used to be a complete workout in itself, depleting me of my remaining energy for the day. Not so anymore!
>
> Twenty-four months ago is when I figured out that I had something I call an "exercise blockage," a sort of invisible

mental funk that has held me back and sabotaged my every attempt to exercise and become healthier.

In my mind, I associated the word "exercise" with pain, fatigue, and numerous failed past attempts at getting into shape. I did not like the word "exercise." Just the sound of the word itself made me tired. So, I shifted my negative self thoughts from losing weight to becoming healthier every day.

I decided to call exercise the Joy of Movement, with all of its grace and the time that I spend doing it—in my case, walking—around in circles inside my house pushing my toddler in his push car with eighties music blaring five to six times a week for forty-five minutes to an hour *Me Time.*

I started (walking) slowly inside my house daily five minutes, then ten minutes at a time. I gradually built up the minutes. Since I live in Michigan and the weather here can be extreme, I needed an activity that I could do inside the house that involved a baby who was quickly becoming a toddler. (Yes, I was blessed with a son, even with fibromyalgia, after three years on the Guaifenesin Protocol.)

At first, I was too fatigued to wear special clothes. Determined to continue my Joy of Movement, I left my nightgown on and just wore my tennis shoes. No sports bra, no fancy shorts. I bought a pedometer to track my success (Omron HJ-112) and held it in my hand. As I progressed, I added more steps and more clothes.

2,500 daily steps over the months evolved into 6,000 steps with a few 10,000 steps here or there. I also added two-pound weights to use every other day. I bought myself a new pair of walking shoes. My first in ten years! I made it routine to immediately put on my Joy of Movement clothes first thing in the morning when I get up, despite how I may be feeling. I am wearing them as I type this now.

> I learned to schedule all of my appointments for the late afternoon, ensuring that I have my special moments to become healthier every day first. Once I put my toddler down for his nap, I soak in the tub and let my muscles relax. I now look forward to my Joy of Movement *Me Time.*
>
> And guess what? I do have more energy. I am losing inches, and I can eat a few things from the liberal side of the hypoglycemic diet and still lose weight!
>
> Chantal in Michigan

## Accomplishing a Goal Each Day

I have found that there is something about having an unmade bed that sort of makes the mind of an already sick person sicker, and that having a made bed sort of tricks the minds of sick people into thinking that they may indeed *not* be sick, if that makes sense.

I decided in my pursuit of wellness that I would indeed make my bed every day. I would make this a part of my daily routine. I would push past my aching muscles and my extreme fatigue, and I would wrestle with my two king-sized comforters, even if it took me all morning to do it. This was my one goal for the day. As pathetic as it may seem, I was determined that this made bed would contribute to my getting better. I reasoned, if my bed is made, then it won't be as inviting for me to remain there for the rest of the day.

Always be thankful for what you are still able to do, even if it is very little when you compare it to your old life and self. Never take for granted what you still have. Friends will come and go, and many healthy family members won't understand you. That is okay. You will meet even better new fibromyalgia / Guaifensin friends who will remain and be able to relate to you. Make sure that you show your appreciation. Remind yourself daily how lucky you are—even on those days when you are feeling crummy. Keep a gratitude journal or recite your blessings daily.

I thank God and the universe every day for the fact that I do not have MS, and that I am still able to see, walk, and hear. And even though it is extremely painful for me to move my body, I still am able to do it. I am thankful for my home and the food that I eat. I am grateful for my friends, my doctors, my family, my husband, my son, my stepson, my cats, my dog, my mother, my father, and my adopted grandfather, Bob.

For me, when I first started the Guai Protocol, accomplishing one goal per day revolved around the hypoglycemic diet. My target for each day was to prepare a hypoglycemic-strict meal for myself and my husband for dinner, with enough for next-day lunch leftovers. I knew that this diet was pivotal in returning me to perfect health. So that was my aim. I kept it simple. I made the meals and then rested the remainder of the day. I let the housework go, because it made my body scream in pain for days. I asked for help, and I enlisted my stepson and husband.

For months, I made preparing nutritious and hypoglycemic-friendly meals my focus. In time, I got my mind back. Gradually I lost weight—forty pounds that first year. I gained more energy. My brain became clearer. My IBS disappeared. My migraines improved. No more nightly potty breaks every fifteen minutes. Gone were the night sweats and the pounding heart. Even if you think you don't need the HG diet, try it. It is extremely beneficial for energy redemption.

Once I felt I had mastered the hypoglycemic-friendly meal preparations, I shifted my focus to one other goal per day, taking a bath. Sometimes I would soak with Epsom salts two or three times per day, because it helped alleviate some of my muscle pain while I remained in the warm water. I always showered afterward to remove the salt, because fibromyalgia can cause you to have very sensitive skin.

Next, I added into my daily routine the goal of getting dressed every day. This did not include putting make-up on, nor did it include blowdryingmy hair. Both of these required too much energy. Holding the hair dryer up over my head was excruciatingly painful and exhausting. In time, I added another component and then another.

Eventually, a few years later, I got to the point where I could take a bath, brush my teeth, blow-dry my hair, and get dressed all at once without ten-minute breaks in between—but still without applying make-up. This daily grooming ritual was usually my only activity for the day. Even if I wasn't leaving the house, I got myself bathed and dressed. It usually took me three hours to complete, but I paced myself.

Because we look normal, healthy individuals simply don't realize how exhausting and completely life-altering having fibromyalgia/chronic fatigue is. They have no idea what it is like to never feel rested or to lie awake all night worrying about the fact that you are going to have to hide, to the outside world, the reality that you did not sleep at all. They have no concept of what it is like to get up for work with the only thought on your mind being when you can return home again to go to bed, where you spend yet another sleepless night staring at the ceiling. They simply can't relate to the fact that our bodies cannot make energy properly and that the simplest task can leave us exhausted for days. All of this is okay. I have made peace with it.

I no longer deplete my energy source by trying to convince non-fibromyalgics or "normals" of the existence of my illness and its multiple afflictions. Instead, I better spend my time creating and practicing more techniques to help me preserve my energy and reclaim my life.

## Visualizing Wellness—More Strategies

I used to believe that I was a great multi-tasker, but what my fibromyalgia and its best friend fibro-fog have taught me is that I am not. The great multi--tasker has left the building. And that, I can now add, is okay. I no longer beat myself up over it. It is what it is, and I am that I am.

I have learned that creating perfect health and becoming well again when you have fibromyalgia involves much more than just taking the Guaifenesin, remaining salicylate-free, keeping a symptom journal, being mapped, and if you are hypoglycemic, following the diet. Yes, becoming well again requires healing our emotions, as well as developing our spiritual side, by learning how to listen to our bodies and understanding what this illness has to teach us.

We all know what the physical aspect of this illness entails for us individually. Each one of us has had to become our own best medical advocate. If you haven't done this yet, now is the time!

Initially, emotionally most of us feel fragile and afraid. Our fibromyalgia/chronic fatigue syndrome has forced us to slow down and unearth things that we never had any interest in finding. Although it was once very frustrating, I can now reflect and see the beauty in it, and one day you will too.

This illness is my greatest teacher. Now that I am in the reversal stage of having and living with fibromyalgia/chronic fatigue syndrome, I view it as one of my life's most sacred blessings. It's forced me to tune in to my body and learn how to take care of my anger and to forgive. It's also sprinkled upon me the healing benefits of what it means to love myself.

Learning to love myself is an ongoing process that takes daily care and effort on my part. To love myself is to put myself first. Putting myself first is a way of conserving my own energy, so I am later able to take care of others. I am not selfish. It is something that my fibromyalgic self needs to do daily, and I have found that it is almost as important to me as the air I breathe. We all need to be kinder to ourselves and to slow down and count our blessings.

Gradually I am learning to do this. I no longer beat myself up by expecting so much of myself. My house, yard, and garden are not perfect, but I am thankful for all of them. I do what I am able to do. When I have visitors, I very gently remind myself that they are here to see me, not my house. In this way, I am learning to love myself. I am accepting the fact that I am that I am right now.

One technique that I practice daily for learning how to love myself is actually a visualization in which you turn the love that you are feeling for someone or something around you inward toward yourself. For example: I feel complete love and a strong, safe connection when I am snuggling on the couch with my husband.

So what I do at that moment is I take that energy, that connection I am feeling with him, and I turn it back into myself. I mentally pull it back into my heart and my being. In that moment, I also take very deep and healing abdominal breaths. I share this energy with myself and with him, and I likewise release any negative self-doubts or thoughts.

It's amazing how energized you can feel when you do this. I use this technique many times throughout my day now with my pets, my toddler, and thoughts that make me happy.

Here is another visualization that I use that keeps me feeling energized. I do this activity sitting or lying down. Very simply, I cross my legs at my ankles and I clasp my hands together in prayer position. With deep abdominal breaths, I envision a glistening white-light energy circulating throughout my body regenerating, starting at my ankles and then coming up my legs and arms, around my head and then down the other side, forming a protective healing cloak around myself. It is my energy armor.

I do this throughout my day; it can be done very subtly. I always do this when I am riding in the car or when I am waiting in the doctor's office. I close my eyes and I do the deep abdominal breathing along with it. Sometimes I combine this exercise with envisioning a huge white bubble around myself, my whole being. This is like a protective shell around me. It helps me focus, relaxes me, and makes me feel safe. I highly recommend *The 10-Minute Stress Manager* audio CD by Emmett Miller, MD, and *Self-Healing* audio CD by Louise Hay, available online at Amazon.com.

While recovering from fibromyalgia, you must stand in your own power and teach yourself how to say *no* to the demands of others around you without feeling guilty. I used to believe that if I were hard on myself, diligent, and disciplined, I would be a better person and that I would somehow become stronger later. I now know differently and silence these mental images. I choose to surround myself with life's vitality and find a balance by saying, "No, thank you, not today."

When I find myself in the midst of negative self-thoughts, becoming overwhelmed or fatigued, I immediately imagine a stop sign in my mind. I use this image to arrest those thoughts and quickly replace them with something more positive and uplifting.

Developing a safe place in my mind through the use of visualization (guided imagery) also helps me empower myself when I am feeling overwhelmed. And believe me, with fibromyalgia, even the simplest tasks can become too much for my central nervous system to bear.

I choose a place in my mind that makes me feel safe, happy, relaxed, and secure. I create everything in my mind for my optimal environment: the location, the climate, the season. I wrap myself up in the smells and the feeling of this safe haven.

I like being on a lake at dusk, floating on a raft tied to a dock, with mountains surrounding me. I reflect on this spot whenever I begin to feel stressed throughout my day. I pull it into the center of my being and let it guide me out of a stressful situation, like a visit to the doctor.

I have always had horrible anxiety about going to the doctor, especially a new one, because I am extremely sensitive to light, sound, and smell. However, I have learned that a couple of meditational techniques for just a few minutes earlier in my day prior to my appointment—usually done first thing in the morning in bed when I wake up—can go a long way.

Again, I start by envisioning the task at hand and then seeing myself doing it successfully, step by step. I view myself in my mind's eye, driving masterfully. I map out my route in my mind. Everything looks peaceful. No construction anywhere. A parking spot near the entrance is waiting for me. I am now in the doctor's office. I am safe, calm, relaxed, and prepared. My visit is triumphant.

I now begin each and every day lying awake in bed for five minutes before I get up. I take this time to listen to my body, and I envision in my mind the major task at hand that I would like to accomplish for the day. I always chose one grand achievement. It could be something like going to see a doctor or going to shop for groceries, both of which take huge amounts of energy for my fibromyalgic self to accomplish. So I take this time to foresee myself being successful.

With deep, slow belly breaths, in through my nose and out through my mouth (to the count of four in and six out), I see myself masterfully carrying out this activity. I envision it to the point that I can see, hear, and feel my surroundings. I stay focused on that one task at hand, and I complete it in my mind, before I even step out of bed in the morning. Once my task is complete, I re-evaluate my energy levels and give myself a huge heart hug and a smile while remembering that *I have fibromyalgia/chronic fatigue syndrome, but it doesn't have me!*

# Part 6

## Reaching Beyond Fibromyalgia

# Chapter 6:
# The Sixth Step: Wanting to Become a Mom

"We must be willing to get rid of the life that we've planned, so as to accept the life that is waiting for us."

—Joseph Campbell

## Fibromyalgic Pregnancy and Motherhood Concerns

"What, you have fibromyalgia? You are too young to have fibromyalgia. Oh, no. You can never have kids with fibromyalgia! If you think that you are nauseated *now* and that you are sick *now,* just wait until you're pregnant. You won't know what hit you. Now, what kind of birth control are you and your husband using?"

"We are using a contraceptive gel, and I am charting my cycle. I know when I am ovulating. We have been using this method for over a year now, since I became sick, and I haven't become pregnant. We are really careful."

"Oh, you will surely become pregnant within this next year, surely. That type of birth control always fails. You can't play around with it. Your husband needs to get a vasectomy right now! He *needs* to get a vasectomy. The procedure is very simple these days for him. He *needs* to get scheduled for one *as soon as possible,* unless you want to become pregnant now. This is serious, and you are so ill. You will become pregnant within this next year, unless he gets a vasectomy. I can guarantee it."

That was my wonderful OB-GYN appointment with a female doctor who shall remain nameless—eight years ago, when my husband and I were both thirty-three years old and in our second year of marriage.

I did not become pregnant within that next year of seeing her. Nor did my husband have a vasectomy. Oh, we debated it. That doctor planted more doubts in my head about fibromyalgic pregnancy and motherhood.

Indeed, eight years ago, I left that well-respected doctor's office shaking, rattled, and nearly in tears. But I never looked back. Instead, I fired her! She clearly wasn't the right doctor for me. However, she does exemplify the typical medical treatment that most of us with fibromyalgia receive. Yes, for every great doctor we encounter, we have to endure—with time, energy, and money— at least two or three lousy ones. She was the second doctor who had advised me against having kids. I have always wanted children but was too afraid to even seriously consider becoming pregnant with the medications that I was still taking.

So when we moved to a new city in August 2005, I met with a new OB-GYN that September. I liked her right away; she was young and energetic. She has a positive out look, and although she wasn't familiar with the Guaifenesin Protocol, she was open-minded about fibromyalgia and assured me that if I wanted to have a baby, there was no reason why I couldn't. It was just best that I do it before age forty. This gave me hope.

> **Note to the Reader:** Reaching beyond fibromyalgia/chronic fatigue syndrome can take on many diverse meanings. For me, after my fibromyalgia "crash," my immediate challenge was going from "bedridden to beyond the futon mattress on our living room floor."
>
> Ultimately, I had three goals: to become well enough to fly from Michigan to California to meet and thank Dr. St. Amand in person; to become well enough to become a mother and experience the joys of first-time motherhood; and to return to full-time employment. Thus far, thanks to the Guaifenesin Protocol, I have completed the first two.

The following passages are excerpts from my personal pregnancy journal, my account of what pregnancy, childbirth, and breastfeeding were like for me after being on the Guaifenesin Protocol for three years. I must add that my pregnancy was an unexpected, yet very welcome blessing.

Please keep in mind that no two pregnancies are the same, even for women who don't have fibromyalgia. However, this is my story. By sharing it, I hope to inspire you. It is not intended to replace the advice of your medical doctor. Always consult your medical practitioner.

For all of you out there who have fibromyalgia/chronic fatigue syndrome and would like to have your own children, but are either too sick or scared to try and/or have been told that you can't birth your own child, never give up. Hope is here. It can be done. I dedicate this chapter to you!

## The First Month

June 20, 2006, Tuesday, Grand Rapids, MI—I am nauseous and dizzy today—more so than just the normal fibromyalgia dizziness and nausea—and I can't understand why. I am spending my day in bed. Josh and I were supposed to go to our first adoption meeting, but Josh doesn't want to. He says that it's too soon after his dad's death. I understand.

June 22, 2006, Thursday, Grand Rapids, MI—Today I decided to start the Restasis prescription eye drops. I need to do something for my dry eyes, even if it blocks my Guafenesin, and it may. I will try to have the drops compounded in a week or so without castor oil in them and then do the blocking test. I don't feel like I am blocking. Usually when I block, I get bladder symptoms—burning and pressure to urinate. I don't have any of those symptoms now.

June 24, 2006, Saturday, Grand Rapids, MI—Josh and Nik are leaving for Vegas today. I'm on house-sitting duty with Kaari, our one-year-old black lab/spaniel mix, and the three cats.

June 26, 2006, Grand Rapids, MI—Michelle is picking me up and we are going to a local department store to buy some baby clothes for a friend of hers who is expecting. The sales were wonderful, so I decided to treat myself and buy $67 worth of clothing for my hope chest—something that I have never done before.

Michelle and I will fly to Canada tomorrow. I hope that I will be well enough for the four-hour flight. I haven't flown in four years, since Mayo Clinic. I will pack protein foods for my blood sugar and plenty of water, just in case.

June 27, 2006, Montreal, Quebec, Canada—The day is here. Food packed and ready to go. I am anxious about flying, yet happy to be going to the mountains once again.

What a day! Our four-hour two-plane flight with connections turned into a twelve-hour misadventure. Ah, Montréal. I am so happy to finally be here!

You've got to be kidding me. Our rental car office is closed? We have to walk—how far? Yes, I can do this! I'm okay despite the fact that it's *HOT* and humid here. My fibromyalgic body can't tolerate the heat or the humidity. It sucks the life force out of me. But I can do this. I am so glad that I packed as much high-protein food and veggies as I did because I sure need them to keep my energy up, head clear, and bitchiness away.

A thunderstorm has just rolled in—a torrential rain, actually—humid and sticky, but we have our rental car and Michelle is ready to drive. She knows Montréal well and is a confident driver.

However, when you can't see the street signs due to the weather, it really doesn't matter how confident of a driver you are. Unfortunately, we are lost, and I need to eat now!

Seriously, with my hypoglycemia, I have major hormonal blood sugar disruptions, and like a diabetic, this can have serious consequences in the moment on my health. Normals simply don't understand the importance of protein and good fats, like olive oil and nuts, to a hypoglycemic, and the urgency in eating every few hours. It's a good thing that I packed as much protein-based food as I did.

This has already been an extremely long day, and we still have another hour and a half's drive north into the mountains after we meet our friends in Montréal. Just in time. Our friends have a nice tuna salad waiting for me and a pizza waiting for my non-hypoglycemic sister.

June 28, 2006, Mont-Tremblant, Quebec, Canada—*Oh, Canada!* How wonderful it is to be here again. I feel happy and virtually pain-free. Yes, virtually pain-free! It must be the mountains and the fresh air. Maybe the change in altitude is easing my pain. No, maybe the Guaifenesin has finally kicked in and I am reversing as anticipated and experiencing a good day. Or maybe I am blocking the effects of the Guaifenesin because of the castor oil in the *Restasis* eye drops. Whatever it is—I feel fantastic—and I am not going to worry about it now!

## Desiring to Become Pregnant

Saturday morning, July 8, 2006, Grand Rapids, MI—Hello, Michigan. I had a wonderful trip, with unexpected spurts of energy, and I could eat foods that normally aggravate my hypoglycemia. It was great to be able to enjoy a few of my favorite oatmeal cookies without consequences. But now it's back to the real world.

I am eight days late. Although I feel like my period is going to start. Since I am normally up to five days late, this isn't alarming me. Not yet, anyway. We always use birth control, and I watch my cycle. But this last time, we didn't, and I was mid-cycle. So we actually could be pregnant.

I mention to Josh that I think I need to take the pregnancy test that is in our bathroom drawer. He flashes me a smirk and kind of laughs. This has been our ritual for the past three years. I have polycystic ovarian syndrome (the number-one cause of infertility in women) in addition to my fibromyalgia, and my cycle can be irregular. I always keep a stash of pregnancy tests on hand. Just in case. Just in case I may need to abruptly stop my medications.

We haven't been trying to get pregnant. But I have been secretly daydreaming. It's my true heart's desire. However, I don't talk about it, for fear that it may never actually happen. I want to become a mom. But I am afraid. Josh and I both want to have more children. But I want to be well enough to care for them. (I have a stepson who is twelve.)

We have a plan, and it's for me to follow the Guaifenesin Protocol for a couple more years and reverse my fibromyalgia as much as possible, re-evaluate, and see how I feel at age thirty-eight. See if I am well enough to even consider getting pregnant. Adoption is also an option for us, but I am concerned that no agency will consider us, since I am unable to work outside of our home. So we are in limbo.

I have made so much progress. I am so happy that I found the Guaifenesin Protocol and the diet for hypoglycemia when I did. The self-empowerment that the diet has given me is fabulous. To be able to stand in my own power: exhilarating. I am a work in progress and thrilled. My advancement is slow yet steady. Every year I keep getting better and better. I have gone from "bedridden to beyond the futon mattress on our living room floor in the dark" in three short years.

However, right now I am smack dab in the middle of making such great progress with the Guaifenesin Protocol that I just can't imagine being pregnant with my fibromyalgia and the chronic fatigue. The thought of stopping and then restarting the Guai is unnerving, since I have no idea how my fibromyalgia is going to react. I dread experiencing a horrible flare and going backwards. I never want to end up on that futon mattress in the middle of our living room floor in the dark ever again. How is my hypoglycemia going to respond? Will I end up with gestational diabetes? And then there is the whole labor and delivery event and a possible C-section. Ugh … How is my fibromyalgic body going to endure?

Sciatica—the pain that extends down my inner thigh from the right buttocks to the arch of my foot—still plagues me daily. How on Earth will pregnancy affect this? Sleep is still my worst enemy, and I don't know how I will survive without my sleep medications. I just can't fathom having to stop my Ambien, Flexeril, or the Guaifenesin. I never thought that I would say that about drugs. But I honestly don't know how I will live without them for nine months.

I guess my fears are legitimate. I mean, I have been so desperate to get well and I have finally found something that works. I have my lifeboat, and I am no longer drowning.

So, our plan is that I will continue to follow the protocol and we will apply for adoption and hopefully welcome a baby into our home by the time we are forty.

I am thirty-six now, and my biological clock is ticking. I know that the longer I am on the Guaifenesin Protocol, the more I will reverse my fibromyalgia and become well. I am torn between the pressure to try to have a baby now or to take the chance to get well enough before we even try.

Dr. St. Amand recommends restarting the Guaifenesin after the sixth month of pregnancy, because the baby will be fully formed and the fibromyalgic mother can also avoid the sudden burst of symptoms that quickly follow delivery. All of this would, however, depend on my OB-GYN and when and if she feels it is okay for me to resume taking the Guaifenesin.

I decide to take the pregnancy test and begin what feels like an eternity of waiting. Suddenly I notice that the pregnancy test box is stamped with an expiration date of March. Ugh … it is now July. My heart begins to race and my face flushes. I am stunned as two solid lines appear. In all of my polycystic-ovary pregnancy-test-taking years, I have never had a positive pregnancy test result, and I can't believe my eyes. I begin to panic and yell for Josh, who notices the expired, but very positive test and knows what needs to be done.

<u>Saturday afternoon, July 8, 2006, Grand Rapids, MI—</u>He returns home with a three-pack. Grin. I am nervous, anxious, yet excited. He remains with me in the bathroom as we take the second test together. Within seconds, two more lines appear. Then the third test, it's another positive!

We decide that we need to share our good news. We bring the tests over to my mom's house and show them to her. At first, she thinks it is a thermometer. She doesn't recognize them because they didn't have home pregnancy tests when she was pregnant with me and my sisters. She can't believe what she is seeing. This is so unexpected. She is overjoyed. We return home and call my mother-in-law, who is in Dallas, Texas, for a doll convention. She is surprised and thrilled. Such joyous news in the midst of such sadness with my father-in-law's recent passing.

Sunday morning bright and early, GR, MI—I spring out of bed with a type of wired, empty energy that is oh so common to my fibroed-out, chronically fatigued body. I am anxious and ready to take the next test. It's our fourth positive test in two days. I can hardly believe it!

Monday morning 9 AM, July 9, 2006, GR, MI—Since I am new to this, I call my internist and request an appointment for an official pregnancy test. (I now know that the home tests are nearly 99 percent accurate and this isn't necessary.) They fit me in for 1:30 PM. It is now 9 AM. My day drags … I can't wait for my appointment.

The doctor's gaze is serious but doesn't allow any clues as to the pregnancy test results. He asks us how long we have been married, and we reply five years this month. He says, "Good, it's about time you have a baby!" Then he proceeds to tell us that I beat the control window. My test changed within thirty seconds. Normally, the test results come back within three or four minutes. Josh and I are delighted—tears of joy!

Josh drops me off at home and he goes to Barnes and Noble Booksellers and buys me the *What to Expect When You're Expecting* books. I dive into them and soon realize that not everything in the book will apply to me, due to my fibromyalgia/chronic fatigue syndrome. In fact, most of it doesn't.

Panic strikes. Immediately, I dig out the book, *The First Year: Fibromyalgia: A Patient-Expert Walks You Through Everything You Need to Learn and Do,* by Claudia Craig Marek, hoping to gain insight about fibromyalgia and pregnancy. It states that many women with fibromyalgia feel better when they become pregnant. That means I may feel better too. Great news, since my own fears are building and my mind is imagining the worst.

I have no idea what to expect during pregnancy—let alone a fibromyalgic pregnancy. I need more literature on fibromyalgia and pregnancy. I search the web and quickly realize that information about fibromyalgia and pregnancy scarcely exists. I am now approaching uncharted waters with my health once again.

Tuesday, July 10, 2006, GR, MI—I stop all of my medications and supplements. This freaks me out, because for three years I have depended on Flexeril and Ambien for sleep. Now without them, how am I going to sleep?

No more Guaifenesin until at least after the sixth month, when the baby is completely formed, if my OB-GYN approves. No more supplements, which include magnesium. I was taking the magnesium for my constipation, hemorrhoids, and migraines. Now what am I going to do?

On the brighter side, I scored a near-perfect when I took the diet self-test in *What to Expect: Eating Well When You're Expecting*. The diet for hypoglycemia that I have been on for the past three years is exactly the diet that is recommended for a healthy pregnancy, and I am psyched!

I decide not to stop using the Restaisis eye drops right away. Instead I put a call in to my eye doctor. I am concerned about the Verapimil for high blood pressure, but I don't stop it either. I put a call in to my OB-GYN's nurse and make an appointment to be seen.

Wednesday, July 11, 2006, GR, MI— Waiting around for the initial OB-GYN appointment feels like another eternity. The pregnancy books all recommend sleeping on your left side. They suggest training yourself ahead of time to sleep on your left side before your bump gets too heavy—usually around the fourth month.

I am a fibromyalgic self-trained back sleeper propped up every night by two pillows—one on each side of me, under each arm—and a bolster under my legs. How am I ever going to learn to sleep on my left side? This new sleeping position is going to be a challenge, but I am up for it.

Insomnia once again has become my nighttime foe without the aid of my muscle relaxants and sleep medications. Although much of my fibromyalgia pain is greatly reduced—thanks to the new pregnancy hormones—I am finding falling asleep without the use of muscle relaxants and sleep aids nearly impossible. I meditate to the best of my ability and wonder how long it is going to take for my body to adjust. I feel wired like my body might be going through muscle relaxant and sleep aid withdrawal. Josh agrees that I need to find a better pillow solution, and he takes me shopping.

Wednesday, July 18, 2006, GR, MI—Even with my two new wedge pillows, large and small, I am still not sleeping. In fact, I have had such terrible shoulder pain for two straight days (one of the symptoms of an ectopic pregnancy) that I tell Josh we need to go to the ER.

Everyone is very kind in the ER. I am seen immediately, and they evaluate my situation. I tell them that I have fibromyalgia, and they ask me if it is neck-, head-, and shoulder-related pain. I answer, "Yes!" The doctor checks my abdomen and my shoulder and sends me on my way with a printout that reads: "Fibromyalgia, Myofascial Pain Syndrome." I am at ease now. The baby is okay. And I am also delighted that they acknowledged my fibromyalgia. A hospital that actually acknowledges fibromyalgia—this is a first for me!

Wednesday, July 25, 2006 GR, MI—Today is our fifth wedding anniversary and I am flat in bed, too nauseous and dizzy to go out to dinner. We order in. I get my favorite pick-three and soon realize that I am too nauseated to eat it. Who said morning sickness was only for the morning? I hope that this doesn't last the full nine months. (I now know vitamin B6 is safe for pregnancy and wonderful for nausea. In fact, it worked so well for me that I continued taking it after pregnancy for my normal nausea associated with my fibromyalgia.)

## The Second Month

Monday, July 31, 2006, GR, MI—Week 8— We had our first ultrasound today—both internally and externally. I am so happy to get a photo of "Peanut Sanders." Although the sex isn't recognizable yet, I feel it is a BOY. My intuition tells me it's a BOY. I know it's a BOY! We will be able to see the sex at the twenty-week ultrasound, and I can't wait.

Sunday, August 6, 2006, GR, MI—I am thrilled to be three weeks away from the second trimester. Rough second month. A lot of dizziness—maybe the blood pressure meds—Aldomet 500mg x 2. Lots of nausea, but no vomiting.

## Preparing for Fibromyalgic Pregnancy

Monday, August 14,-2006, GR, MI—Sleeping position, nausea, and dizziness are my most pressing complaints, and my OB-GYN informed me that these are all normal. That this is pregnancy and it is normal. *That I am normal.* It's spectacular to finally be "normal" again.

However, my most surprisingly annoying and continuous fibromyalgic pregnancy challenge is finding the perfect pregnancy pillow so I am able to comfortably sleep on my left side.

I search the web, read reviews, and decide on a U-shaped full-body pillow. It has gotten excellent critiques for pregnancy and also for fibromyalgia. Unbelievable! A pillow advertised for fibromyalgia. Who would have thought? This truly is the best time to have fibromyalgia.

Thursday, August 17, 2006, GR, MI—My pillow arrives. I welcome it like a long-lost friend. I like it. It cradles me like a baby. But then, after our first night together, I become too hot. And my fibromyalgic body can't stand being hot. "Oh no, now what?"

## The Third Month

Thursday, August 31, 2006, GR, MI—Rough third month; although the baby and I are healthy, I have spent much of my time in bed, on the couch, or in the chair. At times I have been too dizzy, nauseous, and weak to move.

My doctor gently reminds me that this is pregnancy and that I am still normal. I tell my husband that they should rename morning sickness and call it "all day and night sickness." The fantastic part is that I haven't been throwing up at all. Yet I am always "on the verge." So I will remain taking it easy and journal again as soon as I feel up to it.

## The Fourth Month

Tuesday, October 10, 2006, GR, MI—I am feeling better. Better enough to start thinking about when I want to try to get pregnant again after this baby is born. I don't want "Peanut Sanders" to be an only child, since we are having him later in life—although he does have Nik, my step-son, who will be thirteen years his senior when he is born.

Thursday, October 12, 2006, GR, MI—I am up. It is 4 AM. This seems to be my new waking time. I can't sleep or get comfy. I need to write. Here's an update.

I can happily report that being pregnant hasn't been much different for me than having fibromyalgia in its *weakest* form. In general, my fibromyalgia pain has been much improved since I became pregnant. I have not experienced great bouts of fatigue yet. I have more energy, and I actually feel better now that I am pregnant than I did when I wasn't.

Right before I became pregnant, I used to have pain on any given day while reversing with the Guaifenesin in at least twenty-five given areas from head to toe. On a scale of one to ten, with ten being the highest, most of my pain levels ranged daily throughout my body from seven to ten. Now my most painful areas are my neck, head, shoulders (especially my left), and hands. They bother me on a daily basis, with pain levels averaging about three out of ten, with the exception of my left shoulder, whose pain is a ten-plus. This is incredible progress.

With pregnancy, I am noticing that many of my other fibromyalgia symptoms have also improved. My vulvodynia is better, along with my interstitial cystitis (IC.) I am no longer having episodes of burning pain and pressure that feel like a bladder infection every month. My irritable bowel syndrome (IBS) is in check as long as I don't try to eat soda crackers or other carbohydrates for my nausea. I have learned that I can't take the diet advice of normals. They simply don't understand the carbohydrate intolerance and its relationship to irritable bowel syndrome. I start getting abdominal cramps whenever I try to eat a ginger snap or soda cracker.

My headaches are better, but my light sensitivity is worse. My migraines and light sensitivity have always been my worst symptom since I was six years old.

Also, before pregnancy both my sciatica and right hip pain were out of control. Those pains have nearly vanished now. I am shocked at how well the body loosens these muscles to prepare for childbirth. So many of the fears that I had prior to pregnancy I am finding out were just a waste of my time and energy.

I continue to do my physical therapy exercises and tai chi every day. I have added some back strengthening exercises, along with the Kegels. I purchased a prenatal classical compact disc that I love called *Love Chords* by Thomas Verny, MD. I meditate and practice my abdominal breathing daily.

Although sleep has been a problem, it's nothing that I haven't had to deal with in the past with my fibromyalgia/chronic fatigue syndrome. The only difference is, now I am up every two hours using the bathroom and switching from my left to my right side. I have reasoned with myself that this is good preparation for me for when the baby finally arrives and I need to breastfeed every two hours.

My nausea and dizziness have gotten much better. I am able to do more. I spent half of my first trimester moving from couch to bed to chair, due to my nausea. Now, however, in my fourth month of pregnancy, my general pain levels are less, and the areas in my body that are still affected with muscle pain and stiffness are more centralized. It's marvelous! My doctor tells me that the pregnancy hormones are reducing my pain. Why can't we just bottle them up and use them as our treatment?

I can't believe how much time, thought, and energy I have invested in finding the prefect pregnancy pillow. My all-time favorite pillow is the Maternity Pillow by Bean available on Amazon.com. It is carefully designed to support the growing belly and the lower back at the same time. It is made up of two large football-shaped support cushions that are held together by an adjustable Velcro pad. This pad helps you adjust for your personal comfort as your belly grows.

In conjunction with this pillow, I use a five-foot-long body pillow, which I put under my legs while I am sleeping on my side. I alternate between a large and small wedge pillow for my head. These wedges are great for a sore neck and heartburn.

My other favorite pillow is the U-shaped body pillow available online. I know I will love this pillow once the baby is born and I get back to sleeping on my back. It will also be good for breastfeeding in bed. Right now, it is my surrogate sleeping arrangement, and I have it set up on my futon couch downstairs. I found that it is great to use with the couch as back support but wasn't enough support alone for me in bed. It also made me hotter than usual. I use it with the five-foot body pillow between my legs and the small wedge under my head. It's funny, because when I am not using it, I have found my pets enjoying it.

Lately, I have been able to eat a junior ice-cream cone along with a few other carbohydrates without feeling the effects of the hypoglycemia: shakiness, pounding heart, night sweats, and immediate frontal migraine headache pain. I am not sure if this is normal with the new pregnancy hormones or if this is my blood sugar and the fact that I may have already swung into the gestational diabetes category.

My goal for this week is to test my blood sugars with my glucometer and see. I have been enjoying the fact that my hypoglycemia has seemed to quiet down. But I will not push my luck, as I am at high risk for gestational diabetes since I am overweight—a size 14–16 on top and 16–18 on the bottom. I have eaten four kiddy-sized ice-cream cones— vanilla soft-serve dipped in chocolate—since I became pregnant, one ice cream cone a month! This is a huge amount of ice cream for me, since I don't normally eat *any* sugar.

Before pregnancy, my body could not handle sugar at all. For the past five years, my headaches (migraines) would force me to lie flat in a dark room without sound. As soon as I would take a bite of anything sugary, this would be my fate without fail. The left side of my face, under my eye, and in my cheekbone would immediately become numb. The pain would extend down into my jaw and neck. My left eye would feel like a dagger was piercing through it. I would sweat and have heart palpitations. Even a lick of ice cream would ensure night sweats, followed by frequent urination every fifteen to thirty minutes. I was miserable.

Once again, I am astonished at the role diet plays in fibromyalgia/ chronic fatigue syndrome and how so many of my symptoms have been controlled or mitigated by a low-carbohydrate, low-fat diet. Simply superb!

Friday, October 13, 2006, GR MI—Last week, I decided to get up my courage to go to a chiropractor who specializes in adjusting pregnant women. In the past, I have always been afraid of chiropractors. Not so anymore.

The chiropractor worked gently on my neck and left shoulder, which have been out of whack since I started sleeping on my left side. He informed me that the severe shoulder and neck pain that brought me to the ER *three months ago* was actually a dislocated shoulder. Yes, I dislocated my shoulder while trying to train myself to sleep on my left side. I know, only me! My chiropractor popped it back into place for me, and it feels tons better. No wonder I couldn't sleep and finding the perfect pregnancy pillow was such an issue! I also had a half-hour massage by a therapist who has a special chair for pregnant women. She does soft-tissue massage. I am happy to report that for the first time in four years, I was actually *pain-free* in my neck and shoulders for two hours after the massage and adjustment. I will be going back to this doctor's office and recommending maternity adjustments and massages to my fibro friends! (Be sure to consult your regular medical practitioner before starting a new modality.)

## The Fifth Month

Wednesday, October 18, 2006, GR, MI—I have been up since 5 AM and it is now 5:53 AM. I can't sleep due to pain in my arms, wrists, hands, and fingers, and excitement because today is our twenty-week ultrasound and we get to find out the sex of the baby!

Truth be told, I am anxious about having the ultrasound done. Not the actual physical part of the ultrasound being done, but the bladder part and having to drink seventeen to twenty-four ounces of water an hour before the test, with the test then lasting forty-five to sixty minutes. That bladder part makes me nervous, as I have always had an irritable one. I am hoping for the best. I will visualize myself going through this experience and all being well.

Yesterday I went back to the chiropractor. It was my third visit. It really is helping my neck and shoulder, so I will continue to go. My dizziness has been better since he adjusted C1 and C2 in my neck.

I can tell that my hormones are changing once again because my hypoglycemia is starting to become more sensitive. I can no longer eat one corn taco shell without sweating at night or feeling my heart race a bit. I need to buckle down on the diet again. I enjoyed being able to eat my four ice-cream cones during my first four months of pregnancy. The tacos were great too—one per week. I just hope that my hypoglycemia doesn't go into gestational diabetes. But if it does, I am prepared to deal with it.

Today I will also go for my first appointment with a therapist who specializes in EMDR Light Therapy. This treatment is used to reduce stress by releasing trauma from your brain. It has been used for post-traumatic stress syndrome on war veterans. I am hoping that it will help me with my migraines.

Thursday, October 19, 2006, GR, MI—*It's a BOY!* I knew it was going to be a boy ever since the first ultrasound. *I just had a feeling.* This is going to be a bit of a challenge for me, since I was raised in a house full of girls. But I will do fine.

I just pray that he is healthy and on time, not early, and that I don't have to be on bed rest with him. He is ten ounces and his heart rate is 148. I have a low-lying placenta that could move at anytime. I am keeping my fingers crossed that it does. We didn't get to do the 3D ultrasound because he was twisted, but at least we got to see that he *is* indeed a he! I have been calling him a "he" all along—although secretly hoping for a girl. Maybe baby number two will be a girl.

My bladder did just fine through the test. I had to use a lot of mind over matter, because the test took about forty-five minutes and the baby's head is positioned across my bladder on my lower left side. He was sitting Indian style, which made seeing his gender more difficult. But he moved for a second, and the lab technician snapped the picture right in time.

The lab technician also said that my doctor will most likely order a thirty-week ultrasound for me, to check the placenta, spine, and heart again. Since he was twisted, it was hard to see everything. But what she could see looked *good.* I am not looking forward to the thirty-week ultrasound with my bladder issues, but I will put it out of my mind for now and focus on our wellness until then.

Friday, October 20, 2006, GR, MI—It's 2:27 AM. I have decided to get out of bed. I have been up since 1:30 AM and am not able to get back to sleep. If I stay in bed, my body becomes more stiff and full of pain, so I need to get up and do something. I have been registering online for my baby shower. Michelle wants to get my invitations out this weekend. I am hoping that Josh and I will go in person today to scan some items.

Friday, October 20, 2006, GR, MI—My EMDR appointment went very well. I will go back on Monday, and she will begin the protocol for migraine headaches. I am curious to see if it will help, and I am very hopeful. She also mentioned something called energy therapy for treating migraines. It works by using the acupuncture meridians and their connections to the brain.

At this point, as long as it doesn't hurt the baby, I am ready to try anything. In the past four years, I have tried so many different modalities to regain my health—various supplements, visualization, positive affirmations, self-help books and tapes, biofeedback, remote viewing, deep breathing, acupuncture, physical therapy, the Guaifenesin Protocol, a strict low-carbohydrate diet (also know as an anti-Candida diet), reflexology, cranial sacral therapy, tai chi exercises, physical therapy, osteopathic manipulation, foot bath, homeopathy, soft-tissue manipulation, myofascial pain release, trigger-point injections, Botox injections, an activator machine, and now a chiropractor and a massage therapist. I am very thankful for my health insurance and the many incredibly supportive healthcare providers who have assisted me along the way.

I feel that each and every one of these modalities and people has helped me in my recovery. My journey toward wellness has been multi-dimensional: mind, body, and spirit. In many ways, I thank my fibromyalgia for the life lesson that I have learned. I can now say no without feeling guilty, and I am able to ask for help without feeling weak. I've learned to listen to my intuition. My body knows when it is out of balance, and rather than ignoring it, I tune in to it and ask what I need to do to further heal. I am gentle with myself and no longer beat myself up. Each and every day I am thankful for what I am still able to do. I appreciate the little things in life, like the soft purr of my cat, the silky feeling of my bed sheets, and the sweet aroma of cantaloupe as I prepare it. I strive to be in the moment and experience life just as it is. There's no rushing in my world. I have slowed down, and it's a good thing. I've become my own best medical advocate. Vanity and pride no longer lead me. I am not my illness; although I understand I can be changed by it for the better and grow.

<u>Saturday, October, 21, 2006, GR and Grand Haven, MI</u>—Josh and I are going to the pumpkin carving party where we met seven years ago. I am tired, though. The pregnancy fatigue is starting to settle in. We also just found out yesterday that my cat of seventeen and a half years, my college kitty, has kidney failure and she needs IV treatments, a form of kidney dialysis. My mom, sister, and I are to meet at our vet's office later today to learn how to administer the treatments.

<u>Sunday, October 22, 2006, GR, MI</u>—We gave Chelsea her first IV. She is such a sweet kitty, a pure-bred chocolate point Himalayan-Persian with huge blue eyes still full of life and vigor. You would never know how sick she is just by looking at her. She doesn't appear to be in any pain—although I know she must be. I can relate to her—chronic daily pain that is invisible.

<u>Friday, October 27, 2006, GR, MI</u>—Both of my appointments went very well. My OB-GYN gave me the green light to restart the Guaifenesin after my sixth month of pregnancy. I will wait one extra month, just to make sure that the baby is well-formed. She isn't familiar with the Guaifenesin Protocol but seems willing to learn. She also wrote me a prescription for pregnancy hose if I need them.

My eye exam went well too.

Wednesday, November 1, 2006, Grand Haven, MI—I just had my appointment with Dr. Srutwa, my acupuncturist MD and local fibromyalgia miracle worker. My appointment went well. Dr. Srutwa used the myofascial pain release and soft-tissue manipulation on me. I had to lie on my left and right sides for it. No acupuncture due to pregnancy.

Josh drove me because Dr. Srutwa is located an hour away by highway from where we now live. I really miss being able to drive. Someday, hopefully with the help of the Guaifenesin Protocol, I will be able to drive myself long distances once again.

Thursday, November 2, 2006, GR, MI—My EMDR went very well today. I entered her office with a headache and left without one! Still have the pain in my eyes, but it is greatly reduced.

Monday, November 6, 2006, GR, MI—I went to the chiropractor and had a half-hour massage today. I highly recommend these two therapies during pregnancy, but always consult your medical doctor first.

Great news! My chronic fatigue has subsided. I am able to do more now that I am pregnant. I can get up every day, take a shower, get dressed, and dry my hair by 8 AM. This early-morning rising is monumental for me. I still rest while getting dressed, though. But this progress is wonderful. I am also able to nap during the day when needed. My body will relax and fall asleep—something it hasn't been able to do since I was a toddler.

## The Sixth Month

Monday, November 13, 2006, GR, MI—I really don't understand why they don't just say that a woman is pregnant for ten months instead of nine months, considering that we are pregnant for forty weeks, which equates to ten four-week months. I know not all months equate to twenty-eight days; some have thirty-one, and we pick up extra days here and there. But this whole timetable thing is confusing. I am trying to figure out when I will be six months pregnant, so I can restart the Guaifenesin. I can't wait to begin again. Although I have to admit I will miss using mint toothpaste. I kept all of my salicylate-free products the same during pregnancy except mint toothpaste. I decided that it would be much easier restarting the Guaifenesin if I continued using my sal-free products.

My baby shower is a little over a month away. (I have included Baby Registry Must-Haves for the Fibromyalgic Mother-to-Be at the end of this book, as well as shopping tips. We fibro girls have to preserve our energy.

Just figuring out this list can be overwhelming.) Josh has this date as his deadline to get all three rooms painted upstairs. We will be giving the new baby our bedroom and moving into what used to be our office. My sister Nicole should be home from Florida. I will be twenty-eight weeks pregnant. I am planning on restarting the Guaifenesin after week twenty-seven or twenty-eight of pregnancy. I want to make sure that the baby is fully formed when I restart.

I can't believe how fast the time is going now. We will start our Lamaze classes in January.

Saturday, November 18, 2006, GR, MI—I had my monthly Fibromyalgia/Guaifenesin Protocol support group meeting in Grand Haven today. Josh drove me. It went well, and we had a few new fibro patients who are interested in starting the Guaifenesin.

I really enjoy helping people who have fibro and giving them hope. It makes me feel as though my suffering has been worth something. It also shows me and reinforces just how far I have come along, when I work with others newly diagnosed and just starting out on their fibro journeys.

Friday, November 24, 2006, GR, MI—Today I woke up feeling really GOOD! My chiropractor had mentioned to me that by the end of this month, my hormones would be changing again and I should be feeling less muscle pain. He was right. I had energy, and I felt like I had actually slept. I hadn't felt this way in years. I remained in bed and relished in my new found vitality, until the phone rang.

It was my sister, Michelle. She wanted to go to Costco, get her hair cut, and run a few other errands. I needed to get out of the house. So she picked my mom and me up at 1:30 PM. We ran a bunch of errands and we shopped till we almost dropped, but I didn't drop; and I felt pretty good. I hardly hurt, and my headache was the best that it has been in years. We dropped off all items at our individual houses and ended up at Michelle's house for pizza. I ate only the toppings of the pizza and scraped as much of the sauce off as possible, due to its sugar content. At about 8:30 PM, I returned home. I was tired but anxious to get some of my Christmas decorations out. I dug out our small tree and some lights from the basement. Bedtime. What a day, and I kept up with them! This is truly amazing for someone who has fibromyalgia / chronic fatigue syndrome. I feel so great with my fibromyalgia that I am wondering when we should plan to get pregnant with our next baby.

Monday, November 27, 2006, GR, MI—I am finding it truly amazing how my muscles are all loosening up near the end of this sixth month of pregnancy. Wow. My fibro pain is so much BETTER! Although I am finding myself more tired, I am also doing MUCH more. I got all of my Christmas decorations up over the long weekend, even the outdoor ones. I haven't been able to put any decorations up without help for the past four and a half years. This is remarkable.

In EMDR, we focused on changing my fears and concerns about having fibromyalgia and becoming a mother into positive ones—"I am healthy, happy, vibrant, and strong!" I use this affirmation many times throughout my day. I envision myself doing what I want to do without restraint. I also "see" the words as vibrant—in my mind—in human form, sparkling in silver and dancing foot to foot, limbs outstretched, celebrating. This is a wonderful image. It's me, and I am healthy, happy, vibrant, and strong!

## Developing Gestational Diabetes

Thursday, November 30, 2006, GR, MI—Today I have my OB-GYN appointment. Josh won't be able to go with me, so I am a bit nervous about driving myself there. I should be fine, though. I'm not too dizzy. I have my list of questions ready for her. I read that at twenty-eight weeks, they screen you for diabetes by giving you an hour-long glucose tolerance test. I don't want this test. I already know how sugar affects my blood, and I won't put myself through that again. I had my first glucose tolerance test when I was fifteen. It came back negative, although I am truly hypoglycemic and I control it by diet. I was on the long-acting Metformin for six years for my polycystic ovaries. It only brought my twelve-hour fasting blood sugar points down by two when I was on it. That was back in the days before I knew about the low-carbohydrate lifestyle. I stopped it because it made my headaches worse. So I thought.

I have been following the diet for hypoglycemia these past three and a half years now, in order to keep my blood sugar stabilized. I am insulin-resistant and have been for years. For this reason, I will not drink the sugar water.

I am also going to ask her about the metallic/scalded feeling and taste that I have been getting in my mouth. I had this before with the fibro, so maybe it is the fibro again. This week I have also been experiencing some visual stars and vaginal muscular pain—a pulling sensation and then some deep, sharp pains. My sciatica is acting up again too, but that is to be expected as the ligaments along the abdomen are lengthening and preparing for baby to arrive.

Speaking of which, I have been getting some strong kicks and movements from the baby. He is letting me know every day now that he is here and getting ready to see us. I get the feeling that he can't wait to be born. I keep encouraging him to stay in there as long as he needs.

Saturday, December 2, 2006, GR, MI—I am awake! I have been since 3 AM. It is now 4:23 AM. I am *worried.* I had my OB-GYN appointment on Thursday, and everything went well, except for the fact that my doctor wants me to take the glucose tolerance test. I told her that I am hypoglycemic and that I also have insulin resistance. She still wants me to drink the glucose water. I asked for an alternative, as I know how sick I will become for at least two weeks after taking the test. I am *terrified* of this test.

I have taken it before. It always reveals nothing but leaves me with a racing heart, a horrendous migraine, shakiness, irritation, nervousness, aggravation, weakness, nausea, vomiting, impaired memory, confusion, and a feeling of immediate death. No, I won't do this to myself again! But how do I get the doctor to understand me?

This is the predicament many of us with fibromyalgia/chronic fatigue syndrome face. Very few medical professionals understand the depths of this syndrome. We have to become our own best medical advocates, while also being discredited at the same time.

I put a call into Dr. Srutwa yesterday. He knows me, and he knows my case very well. He said that I should not take the glucose tolerance test and that I should try to renegotiate taking another blood test instead. I will call on Monday and talk with my OB-GYN's nurse. I feel absolutely caught in a box.

The fact remains that I am severely hypoglycemic. I know myself and my body. I have been forced the last four years to become acquainted with it. I know what I am like when I eat the wrong foods, and it is not pretty. Even Josh said that I should not drink the sugar water. What the heck, all I ever drink now is plain bottled or tap water. So it just wouldn't make sense for me to drink an orange syrup beverage.

Here I am, up worrying about this and losing sleep over it and putting unwanted stress on *my baby*. Darn it! I have got to get a grip of myself and try to get back to bed. *It will all work out, and you will be okay, Chantal.* I must remind myself that "I am healthy, happy, vibrant, and strong, and I will persevere."

Monday, December 4, 2006, GR, MI—Today was a sad day. We put Chelsea Mae to sleep. Her kidneys just weren't working anymore. My sister and my mom worked diligently for seven weeks with in-home IV fluid treatments, hoping that they would re-stimulate her kidneys. It did not work. I held her as our vet gave her a Demerol shot to relax her before the euthanization.

For the first time in weeks, she looked relieved, and her little kitty body was peaceful. Our vet gave her the final injection. She was gone. I was sad and I felt my throat tighten—making it hard for me to talk. The tears followed next. No more suffering, Chelsea. I will always love and miss you, my little Chelser.

Friday, December 8, 2006, GR, MI—I called today to follow up about the glucose tolerance test. I spoke with the OB nurse yesterday after a day on and off of the phone, and she told me that my alternative method of testing would be to eat ten regular-sized jelly beans one hour before my blood test. I told her that this would not be possible, because once again this was too much sugar for me to ingest. I explained to her that when I eat even two regular jelly beans, my heart races for hours and I sweat and my migraine worsens. I told her that I am really scared to eat those jelly beans and that I even react badly when I eat a bite-sized candy bar. So what other alternative blood test could I take? I told her that I had been tested every three months in the past three years to track my blood sugar. I told her that my doctor ran both the fasting test and the A1C test, and that I am pre-diabetic by typical standards and that I control my blood sugar by following a low-glycemic diet. I am super sugar sensitive, and I can feel when my blood sugar is off.

So, today when I called, I was anxious and nervous and hesitant—but determined. This issue has really thrown me for a loop and shaken my self-empowerment. I have felt the victim once again, for lack of being listened to, believed, and understood. So it took every ounce of courage that I had as I spoke again with the OB-GYN nurse.

She was very kind on the phone and said that I do not have to take that test and that they will consider me as having gestational diabetes. I asked what the protocol would then be for me to follow. How will they know if my pancreas has stopped producing insulin on its own? This is what they told me: I will be sent to a diabetic counselor and given a glucometer. I will test my blood sugar at home eight times a day. I said, "Great! I will do whatever the dietitian tells me to do just as long as I don't have to take the glucose tolerance test ever again."

Friday, December 15, 2006, GR, MI—Yesterday I was feeling really sick—dizzy, weak, nauseous, faint, sweating profusely, salty taste in my mouth—just plain listless.

I had tried to ignore these feelings for the past few days. I had tried to convince myself that I was okay. I had been painting Winnie-the-Pooh characters by hand in the baby's bedroom, trying to get it ready for all to see for my baby shower, which is tomorrow. But, I didn't want to be stupid about these symptoms and ignore something that might be serious.

I decided that I needed to go to the ER after being too weak to hold that paintbrush up and too dizzy to stand any longer. So I called my dad, who is a type-two diabetic, and asked him to bring his glucometer over so I could test my blood sugar. I thought that maybe I had crossed over into the gestational diabetes. My sugar read 93—very good; while his read 163—not so good! It isn't my sugar. That is good. But then the panic hit, and I thought that it must be my blood pressure! So we tested my blood pressure and pulse—both running a bit high.

Everyone was very nice at the ER. It took forever to be seen. They were very short staffed. They retested my blood sugar, which now read 115—still good. I had eaten a couple of almonds and a cheese stick while waiting to be seen. Blood pressure wasn't so high, and there was no protein in the urine. That was a relief! I will follow up today at 1:30 PM with my OB-GYN.

Later Friday afternoon—I am a bit nervous about the visit. Okay, very nervous. For starters, I will be driving myself—something that I rarely do anymore since my fibro crash. The second thing that makes me nervous is her wanting to do the glucose tolerance test. I am scheduled to meet with the diabetes counselor and with the dietitian. I am *not* taking that test! I need to go now and finish painting the baby's room, and then rest and meditate to get ready for my appointment.

My appointment went very well. My doctor says that I am NORMAL! That my concerns are normal and that my tests came back normal! Remember, Chantal—"You and baby are healthy, vibrant, and strong."

## The Seventh Month

Tuesday, December 19, 2006, GR, MI—I met with the diabetic nurse today and with the nutritionist, who told me that I needed to up my daily carbohydrate intake and consider going on medications—not insulin; my blood sugar levels were normal. But simply, she told me that I should go on medications so I could eat whole grains again, to make sure that my body gets all the nutrients it needs from the grains—the grains that make me terribly sick in the first place. She said that I should be able to eat these foods without a problem and not miss out on life—if I am on medications. I just looked at her. (I felt like I had just entered a pissing match with a skunk, but I held my tongue.)

Four and a half years ago, before the protocol, I was bedridden. I couldn't read, think, watch television; my speech was jumbled, and I couldn't care for myself. I sweated all the time; my heart pounded. I had horrible, horrible migraines, irritable bowel syndrome, dizziness, insomnia; all of the symptoms of hypoglycemia. Although all of my blood tests always came back normal, I was *truly* sick. I now know why: I am carbohydrate intolerant.

Dr. St. Amand's diet for hypoglycemia saved my life.

So, now that I am pregnant and my hormones are changing, I will test my blood sugar on the strict diet for a week and then on the liberal diet for a week, watch for symptoms acting up like IBS, and compare the two. If I need to take insulin, I will. I will not, however, take medications in order to eat carbohydrates. That just does not make any sense to me. I will not go backwards!

## The Eighth Month

Thursday, December 28, 2006, GR, MI—We have our regular OB-GYN appointment today. I am nervous again about my morning blood sugar readings. They are averaging 106 but should be less than 100. However, I am testing my blood sugar eight times a day. My numbers are great postprandial (after meals). What I am noticing is that I am feeling shaky, sick, and weak, and extra headachy when blood sugars are reading in the nineties and low one hundreds—the hypoglycemic symptoms at these numbers. This fact makes me really nervous about taking insulin, especially at night, as I don't want to bottom out. I hope that my doctor is going to believe me and understand.

The doctor arrives, and when I explain my findings to her, she agrees with me. I am so happy. I feel heard and understood.

Wednesday, January 3, 2007, GR, MI—We had the ultrasound this morning. All looks well. Baby is weighing in at 3.1 pounds—right on target, which means he isn't getting too much sugar from me. I am so relieved. And although physically I am measuring larger than my expected due date by three centimeters, the baby is actually measuring only four days early. So that is great news. The placenta has also moved away from my cervix and is no longer considered low-lying. I am also very relieved about that. I am just amazed at how lucky I have been throughout this pregnancy, considering how sick I was for the past four and a half years. I just feel so lucky and blessed and happy. Had I known that pregnancy was going to be like this, I might have tried it sooner!

Thursday, January 4, 2007, GR, MI—Josh and I went to our breastfeeding class. He was the only male there. Ha ha!

The class was long—almost three hours—and boring. I would not do it again. I learned a bit, but it was hard to concentrate. The television in the room had a very loud buzz to it that my fibromyalgic self couldn't block out.

It's times like these that make having fibromyalgia completely debilitating. Between the fluorescent lighting and the harsh hissing sound of the television, I was miserable. I wore my sunglasses and a large hat, because for now I can't function without them. The longer we sat there, my headache kept getting progressively worse and worse. I felt very nauseated and in pain. Finally at break time, I asked the instructor if she could turn the television off, since she also had a large display screen that she was using and the class was small. She said that she would, because the buzzing was also upsetting her hearing aids. Imagine that!

I have to be honest here. I don't know if I will be able to attend the Lamaze classes. They will also be held in that room. I don't know what I am going to do if that loud buzzing noise returns. I told Josh that we should get there early so we can pick a good seat away from the television. I might also bring earplugs and muster up enough courage to talk to the instructor beforehand and ask if he or she is planning on using the television. One thing that having fibromyalgia has taught me to do is stand up for myself. So we will see. The important part is that I don't waste too much time worrying about the class. Josh also has told me that if it is miserable, we will leave. What will be will be. I can only do my best.

Monday, January 8, 2007, GR, MI—I can't believe that I have only eight weeks until the baby is born. Incredible! Almost everything is ready for him. Our bags are packed for the hospital.

Our Lamaze classes start tonight. I need to gather up two pillows, a blanket, and a doll and keep a very positive attitude.

I also have to decide when I am going to restart the Guaifenesin. Sometime this week, I think. I am a bit nervous about it. I am starting to feel the extra weight as I lie on my side. But other than that, I can't complain. I went to the chiropractor on Friday for an adjustment. The adjustments are really helping. I highly recommend them. Also, my pregnancy pillow is wonderful. I would be completely uncomfortable without it. I still do my tai chi, physical therapy exercises, and Kegels every day and highly recommend them too. Although I have to say, if I could bottle my pregnancy hormones and take them for the rest of my life, I would be happy. They have really helped my muscle pain.

Tuesday, January 9, 2007, GR, MI—Today is my baby sister Mippy's birthday. Happy thirty-first, Michelle!

We had our first Lamaze expectant parenting class last night. I packed my nuts and cheese stick and water. The class was almost three hours long, with a lot of matt work. I was sore afterward, but not terribly. Thank you, pregnancy hormones.

We were the oldest couple there, and I was the only one wearing sunglasses and a hat. At thirty-seven years old and teary-eyed, I feel very blessed to be having my first baby. Every day I thank God and the universe for this opportunity and for the little treasure growing inside of me!

Having fibromyalgia and being pregnant is not easy, but having fibromyalgia and being pregnant with a purpose makes it all worthwhile. I have had many days where I have felt better being pregnant with fibro than with just having the fibro. I am fortunate. My migraines have improved somewhat. My pain levels are generally lower on a daily basis.

I had to laugh when I heard the Lamaze instructor ask for a show of hands on how many of us moms-to-be have backaches, nausea, heartburn, fatigue, and difficulty sleeping. These are just a few of the symptoms of fibromyalgia that I live with daily when I'm *not* pregnant. I think having fibromyalgia has actually prepared me in these ways for pregnancy. So, if you have fibromyalgia and you really want to become a mom—go for it! Follow your heart and intuition (and always check with your doctor).

Last night at bedtime, after the Lamaze class, I decided to take the plunge and restart the Guaifenesin. I am due in exactly eight weeks. My cycling dose pre-pregnancy was 300 mg times two. I took 300 mg last night, and today I am not feeling too different—a big change from when I first started Guaifenesin on August 14, 2003.

Thursday, January 11, 2007, GR, MI—Today I am feeling the effects of restarting the Guaifenesin in my mood. Yesterday, I was irritated and "down" with a terrible headache in my right eye, jaw, top of my head, back of my head, neck, and shoulders. I was miserable. This is to be expected. My body is going through yet more changes with the Guaifenesin. I spent most of my day in my La-Z-Boy chair, and I am at peace with it.

Today I am a bit better. I need to call the chiropractor and get in with him. Josh and I have a baby class tonight, but we have both decided that we are going to skip it. It's in the same room as the Lamaze and breastfeeding classes, and quite honestly, I can't tolerate the environment tonight after restarting the Guai.

I can't believe how much money I have spent on plus-sized maternity bras, tank tops, and underwear. I was a size 14-16 top and a size 16-18 bottom when I became pregnant. This has been one of the most challenging aspects of pregnancy for me. I don't know how even-larger women do it! I finally found underwear and tank bras that fit online.

Sunday January 14, 2007, GR, MI- Today my pain levels are all very low—around a three except for my right calf that has been bothering me since Friday. The chiropractor tried to stretch it for me and he used the activator on it, but it didn't help too much. He also taught me some new stretches, but still nothing is helping. I used to get trigger point injections in this area before pregnancy, but stopped once I found out that I was pregnant.

Today has been a weird day. I got up, took a shower, and decided not to get dressed. I haven't done much of anything. I talked to a few friends on the phone and just relaxed. My pain levels are so low that I have forgotten that I am pregnant—except for my calf. It hurts so much I could cry. I will try to soak it in some warm water.

One thing that I am really noticing since restarting the Guai is how my urine smells—so strong. This is a really good sign as it must be the calcium phosphate purging out of my system once again.

## The Ninth Month

Friday, January 19, 2007, GR, MI- My OB-GYN appointment went very well. No ketones or protein in my urine. Great! I am super happy about that. Thank you, God and the Universe. "I am healthy, vibrant, and strong. Alexander and I are healthy, vibrant, and strong!" My OB-GYN said that the baby is considered full-term anytime after 37 weeks, but if my water broke at 34 weeks she would deliver and he would be fine. I can't believe that I am already measuring at 34 weeks. I hope that he stays in there as *long* as he needs to, as long as he doesn't go past the 40 weeks, that is! I want him to be in top form when he is born.

Sunday, January 21, 2007, GR, MI- I do have to admit that this week has been a horrendous one for my migraines. I really miss going to acupuncture weekly and getting soft-tissue manipulation. My blood sugar is testing normal so I know that isn't it. It must be a combination of the weather—we have had many storms here in Michigan as winter has finally hit this week, my pregnancy hormones must be changing again, and I think, also, that it is restarting the Guaifenesin that is putting more shock and strain on my muscles. I am going to try to get in with the chiropractor tomorrow before Lamaze class, otherwise, I am afraid that the class is going to be too much for me to sit through for nearly three hours! I have been in terrible pain with my right shoulder, neck, head, and right arm. I started using my water pillow for my head again last night. I used to use it pre-pregnancy when I slept on my back.

Sunday January 28, 2007, GR, MI—We celebrated my dad's seventy-fourth birthday last night by going out to dinner and then over to his house for a party with his friends. I didn't eat even a bite of cake or ice cream. I have been noticing that my morning blood sugar readings have been slightly elevated—not every morning, but a handful of them since I restarted the Guai. I don't know if there is a correlation or if it is just the fact that I am in my *last* and hopefully *final* month of pregnancy now. I say this because I have heard of many fibro women delivering ten-month babies. I am praying that this won't be my case. I feel positively that it won't.

I have been up since around 5 AM. I have a very stuffy nose today and a sore throat, along with very dry eyes. I couldn't sleep because I was hungry. Now I am feeling shaky and weak. I took my blood sugar again, and it looks fine. I think that it's my pregnancy hormones and lack of sleep. I will go this Thursday to the OB-GYN, and I will ask her about my blood sugar readings. I also dropped my monitor by accident. I called the company to see if I could get a new one, and they had me run a systems check on it. They felt that it was still accurate despite the fall. I will ask my doctor about this and then follow up on it with the company. I also need to start taking my blood pressure at home to watch for the pre-eclampsia. I have tightened up my diet and made it as salt-free as possible. I allow myself only two salted cashews a day—the rest of my nuts are either almonds, walnuts, or natural salt-free peanut butter with an occasional salt-free peanut.

My weight gain has been twenty-seven pounds to date. One week I actually lost two pounds. I really don't want to gain more, for a number of reasons, mainly my blood pressure.

I can say that fibro aside, the single most difficult thing about my pregnancy has been finding undergarments that fit. Who would have thought? I went from a 44-D to a 44-DDD. I finally found a nursing bra, Bravado Double Support, that fits me now, with one month to go. I have read that my breasts may increase yet another size once my milk comes in. I do have to say, though, that I really like the way my body looks, pregnant and naked. "I am woman, hear me roar!"

Underwear that is comfy and fits right has been another Internet adventure for me. I always wore Hanes Her Way High-Cut Briefs. I don't like anything tight around my legs or anything that doesn't completely cover my derrière. After tons of trial and error, I finally found all-cotton high-cut briefs online.

## Waiting for Baby

Wednesday, February 8, 2007, GR, MI—Today was exciting. Not only is it my dad's actual birthday, but it also was my first time to go to the ER for false labor. I have been having the Braxton-Hicks contractions off and on all day. At first it was no big deal, but by 2:30 PM I had one that doubled me over, took my breath away, and seemed to last for an hour and a half! I called the doctor, and they said to go in to the ER just in case.

Mippy and my mom took me. Everything checked out okay. Urine looked good. Contractions showed up on the monitor, and they gave me some IV fluids to help with the pain. I was released about three hours later.

I am glad that I went to the ER and that everything looked fine. That put my mind at ease.

Tuesday, February 13, 2007, GR, MI—Twenty-three days left! Just about three weeks. The countdown has begun. I am converting my fear of delivering into "Welcome home, baby." I want him here with us.

Sleep is becoming nearly impossible now, with my head, neck, and shoulder issues with the fibro. I have gained thirty pounds, and although I am thrilled by this amount, it is sure putting a strain on my body, mainly on my ribcage at night and my lower abdominals. I also feel it in my arms and legs when I try to prop myself up and out of bed to go to the bathroom every two hours. Ah, the wonders and joys of pregnancy! Will I ever do this again?

Today I have more heartburn and a very stiff and sore neck and shoulders. The muscles across my right breast are also very tender and burning. I tell myself, "We are healthy, vibrant, and strong." I hold on to this thought; solidify it in my mind.

To my husband's dismay, I decided to wear disposable undergarments to bed last night. I felt more confident wearing these pants, although I didn't need to use them. Just knowing that I was covered was a comfort. I also feel more confident in case my water breaks. This getting up every two hours to go to the bathroom is annoying. It's easy at this stage in pregnancy for me to sneeze or cough and have a leak, despite all of the Kegels.

Everyone tells me that it looks like the baby is lower—like he is dropping. Sometimes I feel like he has. Although, last week in the ER, he looked like he hadn't dropped yet. We will go this Thursday to the OB-GYN, and she will check then to see if he has dropped.

I do have to add here that despite all of the pain I have been feeling lately, it is nothing like the pain I have experienced with just the fibro. Being pregnant and having fibro has been so much better than just having fibromyalgia.

I feel like the luckiest girl in the world. I am so blessed to be able to be having this baby. Words can't describe how happy I am. I had planned on adopting and still would like to someday. However, being able to go through this pregnancy journey has been incredible.

Feeling the baby kick inside of me is something that I could never have imagined. It's amazing to have this little miracle inside of me. Every time I go to an appointment and my urine checks out fine, I envision in my mind's eye running a relay race. I am being passed this red, white, and blue baton. It is glowing, and I am leaping with huge strides and running so effortlessly, I am nearly floating through the air. I can breathe very well. My asthma isn't bothering me at all. I feel very exhilarated and happy and free. "I am almost there. We are almost there! *I am no longer waiting for the flood.*"

Seeing my naked, pregnant form is really something, too. I can say that I really like my body pregnant. For the first time in my life, I really like my body, stretch marks and all. I am hoping that this new admiration for my body will last once the baby is born. I don't want to beat myself up over my weight anymore.

Thursday, February 15, 2007, GR, MI—I went for my OB-GYN appointment, and she said that I was 50 percent effaced and one centimeter dilated. I asked her what that meant exactly, and she said that for a first-time mother, that is good. It means that my cervix is starting to change and that the baby is getting in position to move out. She said it could take a day or a week or two. Not at all like the movies. So I have been keeping track of my contractions and waiting.

Sunday, February 18, 2007, GR, MI—I had a really good day today, and I just got ready for bed and noticed that the baby has dropped. I was feeling more pressure than usual and a pulling in my loins. Now I understand why. How exciting.

Wednesday, February 21, 2007, GR, MI—Wow, this kid is keeping me on my toes! He keeps testing the water and giving me three- to five-minute-long contractions for an hour or so, and then they taper off! I called the OB-GYN nurse, and she said that this is normal. She also said that the contractions will get so strong that I won't be able to talk. I got a taste of that yesterday, but still no baby. I have to keep reminding myself that he will come when he is ready.

Thursday, February 22, 2007, GR, MI—I am feeling pretty well today. I will have Josh take me to the chiropractor when he comes home after school.

Friday, February 23, 2007, GR, MI—Josh is hoping that the baby will come on his birthday, February 24. That means that I would have to start my labor today. I have had the feeling all along that he will come early or at least before his due date of March 8, 2007.

Saturday, February 24, 2007, GR, MI—Happy birthday, Josh! We decided to go ahead with his party. Everyone is coming over tonight for pizza and cake.

At around 8:00 in the evening, I started having contractions that were three minutes apart, and my blood pressure was high, but not high enough to deliver the baby via C-section. It was hard to know if I should go to the hospital or not. The contractions lasted for an hour. I was instructed to lie on my left side and count them. Everyone was waiting to see if the baby was going to come. They had never been to a birthday party quite like this. Anticipation and excitement filled the air. After an hour and a half, my contractions stopped. No baby tonight. They must have been Braxton-Hicks contractions. It's so hard to know, when this is your first baby.

Sunday, February 25, 2007, GR, MI—Still no baby!

Monday, February 26, 2007, GR, MI—Emergency ultrasound at my OB-GYN's office to make sure that there is no fetal distress, as my blood pressure has been elevated.

Tuesday, February 27, 2007, GR, MI—We met with my OB-GYN at her office to talk about being scheduled for an induction. I am now officially pre-eclamptic. They have found protein in my urine, and my blood pressure is spiking. Thank you, God and the universe that this is happening *now* in the final week of my pregnancy. Thank you for holding off and giving me an otherwise healthy and vibrant pregnancy.

I am scheduled for an induction on Thursday morning at 6:00. I am to be at the hospital March 1, at 6 AM. Our baby is finally coming!

## Welcoming Alexander Neil

Wednesday, February 28, 2007, GR, MI—This was by far the most joyous day of my life! I accomplished the impossible today. After only three short years of being on the Guaifenesin Protocol, Alexander Neil Sanders emerged into this world happy and healthy. Here are the details:

I woke up for my usual every-two-hour pregnancy potty break. It was 1:15 Wednesday morning. I always rest for a few minutes when getting up from a reclining pose, to make sure that my blood pressure is stabilized, because I don't want to fall.

Suddenly, I felt an urgency to urinate with lots of pressure, but I was tired, so I lingered longer before getting up. I was sleeping downstairs on the futon sofa, where I have been for a few months now. I found it easier to sleep on my left side with back support from my pregnancy pillow this way, and I also didn't want to wake Josh up with my frequent potty breaks.

I decided to inch myself slowly forward and off of the mattress. As I did this, I immediately felt the huge gush of fluids. It was a never-ending rush of warm, sticky water and then a steady trickle. I tried to hold my bladder, but it still kept coming. *Did I just wet myself?*

"Josh!" I yelled from downstairs as I realized what just happened. "My water just broke!" I didn't want to move for fear that I would damage my pregnancy pillows and bedding.

Meanwhile, Josh responded with a simple, "Okay, I'll call a substitute teacher to take my classes for tomorrow," and then I heard a whole lot of stomping and scampering upstairs. I yelled to him to bring me a disposable undergarment. In a flash, he was standing before me, dazed when he saw all of the water.

I managed to put my most prized pregnancy pillow between my legs, and he helped me waddle to the bathroom. The water kept coming. The sanitary pad that I had been wearing didn't hold any of the liquid. I was soaked. I managed to put on one of the disposable undergarments. It held the fluid very well.

It was winter in Michigan, and the roads were super icy. We were in the midst of a winter storm and on our way to the hospital. Thank goodness we only live a few minutes away.

The drive to the emergency room was very bumpy, and with every bump, more liquid gushed. Many thoughts were running through my head, my main thought being: *I guess I won't be having an induction tomorrow at 6 AM after all. It feels like the baby is coming now!* I practiced my breathing exercises and tried not to push. The rectal/vaginal pressure was starting to build. I reminded myself that I couldn't push quite yet. I didn't want to damage the baby. I wasn't feeling strong contractions, yet the water was still coming. *I couldn't believe how much water there was. It was warm and sticky—a foreign feeling. I was glad that I was wearing the disposable undergarment.*

I was wondering how I was going to get out of the car and walk into the hospital, I feared being soaked and making a huge mess.

Josh dropped me off at the emergency entrance. The attendant saw that I needed help, and he quickly brought me a wheelchair. They recognized me in the triage area. Everyone was very kind. I was slightly nervous and anxious about when this baby was actually going to come. At least I was now in the right place.

They quickly moved me up to the OB ward and into the first OB triage room. They confirmed that the fluid was indeed amniotic when it turned blue immediately. I was sent into my own private labor-and-delivery room, located across from the nurses' station.

I was hungry, tired, desperate, and drained. The past five days of emergency room visits and anticipation had really worn me out. I wanted to eat something. It had been a few hours since I had eaten anything, and my hypoglycemia was starting to roar. I asked if I could eat a cheese stick. I explained my situation. The nurses said no. They didn't understand nor did they care about my situation with my blood sugar. I didn't know how I was going to survive without some food—more exactly, protein. So I tried again and I asked if I could drink some of my whey protein powder. "You may have ice chips." How about having some ice chips mixed with protein powder? "No."

The doctor came in to check me. I was dilated to four centimeters and 75 percent effaced (cervix softened). I needed to be dilated to ten centimeters for the baby to come. No hard pushing was allowed until ten centimeters. I decided that I wanted an epidural when the time was right. They told me that I would do something called "laboring down." Once I received the epidural, I would let the epidural do the work for me and move the baby down the birth canal. I would do very soft grunt pushing, and I would remain in the bed on my left side. I have high blood pressure, and this is one way to control it.

I met my nurse and asked her if I could have an enema. I have never had one before, but we had learned in our Lamaze class that this would be possible, and I really needed it. I hadn't had a bowel movement in three days. Constipation is very common for me, aside from pregnancy.

My nurse told me that what I was feeling was the urge to push the baby. I assured her that it wasn't. She told me that they no longer give enemas before birth. Even though I hadn't been in labor before, I knew my body. This was constipation. I was so uncomfortable that I had to get up and go into the bathroom to try to go. Nothing happened. I was worried that I would push too hard too soon. I was so uncomfortable; it was hard to breathe, sit, lie down, or stand. The contractions were coming steadily, yet I knew that I had to have a bowel movement. So I got up and I held on to the safety bar in the bathroom, next to the toilet. It was cold and it felt good. I was hot and in extreme pain from the constipation. The contractions came and went, and I could breathe through them. I realized in that moment that the pain of childbirth wasn't as bad as the chronic daily pain of living with fibromyalgia. I was comforted by the fact that I knew my contractions would ebb and flow. Still holding the bathroom bar, I swayed back and forth. I tried to bend a bit, to force my bowels to work. They didn't. I was so uncomfortable at this point I didn't know what to do with myself. I got back in the bed. Once there I got on my left side and realized that I needed to get up again. I returned to the bar in the bathroom, and I continued to sway back and forth. My stomach was cramped, and I knew that my constipation was making these contractions worse.

After a few hours, a hospital work shift change occurred, and I got a new nurse. I desperately asked her if I could have an enema. I explained to her my situation in great detail—too detailed to share here.

She told me that she would see what the doctor could do. She returned with the enema. I was embarrassed but desperate. She told me to "let it rip." I was on my left side in the bed with padded removable sheets under me. I let it rip and realized how awkward the situation was. I mean, letting it rip in front of this nurse, my mom, and my sister. (My husband was glad that he was downstairs eating breakfast with my dad and missed it.)

But I did it and I felt better—much better. I liked this lady. She had a wonderful way of calming me down and putting me at ease. I was glad that she was going to be my delivery nurse. They checked to see how dilated I was. I was now an eight! The nurse called the anesthesiologist, and everything happened very fast. Everyone raced around, and I felt their urgency. The epidural was coming, and if I didn't get it now, I would miss my window of opportunity.

The epidural really helped lower my blood pressure. I had been very concerned about what my blood pressure would do during labor. Now I knew.

The epidural seemed to take the edge off of the contractions. The contractions came and went. They were strong and sharp. I started my abdominal breathing and put myself in another place. "Focus on your breath," I gently told myself. "Focus on your breath. Flow with the contractions. See yourself gently riding the waves. Imagine yourself floating on the lake at dusk in the mountains on the air mattress." A few more hours passed. The time was going by quickly for me. But I was becoming more and more exhausted with each passing hour.

The baby was just not coming out. His shoulders were too big, due to my gestational diabetes. He was also too low in the birth canal to do a C-section. They suggested using the forceps but were concerned that his shoulders would get stuck. The doctors and the nurses, all six of them, went out into the hallway to discuss my case. My mom and sister became worried. My neck was throbbing in pain and stiff from all of the pushing. My headache was fine, and my hypoglycemia had seemed to reset itself. I was wearing my sunglasses and my bite splint. My TMJ was also fine. Thank God and the universe. But I was exhausted, and the pushing was now growing old. It had been two hours of heavy pushing and eleven and a half hours of active labor. The doctors returned with a sheet, and I was to put my feet into some stirrups and pull myself up from my reclined position. My fibromyalgic body rebelled and the throbbing in my arms began. I was too tired to pull, but I tried my best. It was not working. The baby was fine. He was not in distress at all, but I was. I was tired and losing more and more energy. The fatigue was almost overcoming me. But I wouldn't allow it. "I must get this baby out," I silently told myself.

The doctors brought in a contraption that resembled a football goalpost. They attached it to the end of my bed. I was to squat and straddle it with my arms and push with my contractions, but my contractions weren't coming fast enough, and this made me become even more exhausted. I was certainly glad that I had only gained thirty-four pounds. I was becoming more and more frustrated. I could see what looked like the top of his head crowning. It looked like he wanted to come out, but he was stuck—really stuck.

I focused on my breathing, and then my mom stepped in and held my neck up. She started to tell me that I really needed to concentrate and to push that baby out. "You need to push him out right now!" Josh stepped in and started to count aloud, and this helped me. The doctors gave me Pitocin, and my contractions came faster, and this was finally the extra help that I needed.

But the baby still didn't emerge. I wanted him out and here with me. I wanted him healthy and alive here with us! My mom encouraged me and held the back of my neck up for me. It was sore and I needed the extra support. Josh counted and coached me. His voice became louder and more encouraging. Finally I saw hair and head emerging. I thought it was his whole head, but it wasn't. It was only part of his head. No wonder he wouldn't come out. He was huge!

Finally, I gave it my all. I closed my eyes and bore down hard until I felt this squishy painful tightness in my vagina and then my stomach deflated like a beach ball. I listened for a cry, but I didn't hear one. So I yelled, "Speak, baby, speak! Breathe!" And then, relieved, I heard it, a faint little cry—not ferocious at all like I had imagined, but a sweet little "Wah."

The doctors rushed him away from me, and they did all of the Apgar testing. They also realized that his blood sugar was very low, due to my gestational diabetes, and they took him to treat him. The nurses brought him back and put him on my chest. He was beautiful. I was filled with awe and a deep sense of relief.

I couldn't believe that he was finally here with me, with us, after twelve hours of labor and two and a half hours of hard pushing. It was 1:22 PM, exactly twelve hours after my water broke. On Wednesday, February 28, 2007 we welcomed, Alexander Neil, nine pounds, six ounces, and twenty-two and a half inches long into this world. The nurse helped me latch him on my breast, and he began to feed peacefully.

## Hoping to Breastfeed

The lactation consultants immediately streamed in, one after another. Each one was pushy and bossy, and I became stressed. My orders were to feed him right away without delay. Very busily they fluttered around the room, flicked the lights on, and opened the blinds without even thinking that the lights might have been off for a reason.

I was the reason. My migraines and light sensitivity were the reason. I can't function under fluorescent lights. Those lights are death to me—I hear them buzzing and see them flickering, and they rapidly induce my migraines. Seriously, this lactation consultant was acting like it was all about her. Stressed, my milk suddenly didn't flow. My milk had been flowing a few minutes earlier and everything was fine. The baby had had a great latch-on, and he was slurping away as happily and as calmly as could be. Not so anymore.

When the nurse came in to check on me, at first glance she immediately knew something was very wrong. I had gone from overjoyed to annoyed, in a few short minutes, even panicked, and I was sweating. I explained to her what had happened, and with her help, I fired those lactation consultants.

Luckily for me, all of the nurses had been trained in breastfeeding, and they calmly helped me one by one, around the clock. They were wonderful, and they made me feel at ease. They also told me that I didn't seem like a first-time breast-feeder. This made me feel good.

We focused on the football hold, and I practiced it each time they brought the baby in to me throughout the night. Alexander had to stay with the nurses and be bottle fed due to his low blood sugar. I actually felt relieved to know that he was safe with them, and for the first time since my water broke, I tried to sleep.

I was wired, and I couldn't sleep. Post-partum anxiety had silently crept in. I was sure that it wasn't my blood sugar, because I had ordered a steak and green beans and had eaten them after Alexander's first feeding. Since the diet for hypoglycemia is vital for my well being, I made sure that I followed it exactly as written, especially here in the hospital. I concluded that my anxiety wasn't food related this time and decided to request an Ambien for sleep. It was now 3:00 in the morning and I really needed to sleep.

The next day, my vagina, where I tore during delivery, was terribly sore, and I was bleeding like crazy. I was told that all of this was very normal. Once again, I was normal! My mind was at ease but amazed at what the pregnancy books chose to omit. They neglected to mention that breastfeeding the baby could take up to two hours at a time, due to the baby's hiccups and gas. Craziness, since he needed to be fed every two hours! But newborn babies do indeed get gas and they do get the hiccups—hiccups that can last for hours. And it's all completely normal.

I have decided to be in the moment each and every time I nurse him, no matter how exhausted I may be. I want my milk to flow and my baby to be calm and relaxed.

I am making a conscious effort to begin my breastfeeding journey without placing any expectations on myself. I know that this time is a sacred time for me and my baby. Everything else can wait. Mommy and baby need to bond. I remind myself that we are both learning and that in the beginning, breastfeeding takes practice and patience. We will *both* get the hang of it. I have decided that I am not leaving the hospital until I feel that I have mastered the football hold. I remain calm.

Breastfeeding is natural. I concentrate only on the task at hand. I focus on my breath. Breathe. I listen to the little sucking sounds that my baby is making. I focus on the love, nourishment, and support that I am providing him. I am gentle with myself.

Thursday, March 1, 2007, GR, MI—Breastfeeding is going very well. I am using the Boppy and hoping that my fibromyalgia won't flare. So far it hasn't, and I feel great. I restarted the Guaifenesin two months prior to delivery. The nurses are very supportive and patient with me. I am happy. Alexander is beautiful. He is no longer a floppy baby. Thank God and the universe! Everything seems surreal in a very good way. I have had a stream of visitors and much love and support coming through my door all day. We get to leave the hospital tomorrow. Motherhood is awesome, and I want to shout out and proclaim to the world, "I have fibromyalgia/chronic fatigue syndrome, but it doesn't have me!"

# Afterword: Meeting Dr. St. Amand for the First Time

"The years teach us much which the days never knew."
—Ralph Waldo Emerson

## Flying to Los Angeles, California

Five years. Five years and I am finally here at the airport, headed for Los Angeles, California, to meet and thank Dr. St. Amand, the man who gave me back my life. I can't believe it. I have worked so hard for this moment.

Saturday, June 7, 2008, GR, MI—It is noon. My sister Michelle, nicknamed Mippy, is my travel buddy. We are traveling to be seen by Dr. St. Amand on Monday morning. Our flight leaves Grand Rapids today at 2 PM. I can hardly wait.

We arrive in Minneapolis with three hours to spare before our next flight. Just enough time to get some lunch and people-watch. Things are looking up, and we are both excited.

We have arranged to meet a friend of ours tomorrow named Sam, who is ninety-three years young and still lives in his own home in Cerritos, California, just thirty minutes outside of Marina del Rey. We met Sam and his wife Ida on a bus tour of Europe pre-fibromyalgia crash for me in 2001. Both in their eighties, Sam and Ida practically led the tour with their vitality for life and endearment for one another. I am looking forward to seeing Sam again and so sorry to hear about Ida, who recently passed away.

It's announced that for mechanical reasons, our flight is delayed an hour coming into Minneapolis. That is okay. An hour is not too long to wait. I do, however, have to note that flying when you are hypoglycemic is totally doable, but it involves more planning.

I always pack Solgar low-carb whey protein powder. I keep it in a Munchkin plastic toddler snack container, which has a spout and divided sections. It's perfect for pouring into an empty water bottle and then mixing with water after going through airport security. Cheese sticks, packets of tuna, chicken, celery, an apple, and homemade trail mix consisting of walnuts, almonds, peanuts, and sugar-free coconut all go into my carry-on luggage. I attach a small cooler to my purse. It's actually made to hold a baby bottle, and it is insulated, made by JJ Cole available at Target online. Boy, am I happy that I planned ahead.

We board the plane and remain on the runway for three hours without air conditioning. It's announced that the plane now has two mechanical problems. My sister and I are relieved that the problems were caught and fixed, however it is now nearly midnight. We have been traveling since noon Michigan time. More disturbing news—the crew has exceeded their sixteen-hour workday, and they need to call in another crew. That means more time on the runway for us.

I begin to sweat. I feel faint. Heat doesn't agree with my fibromyalgia. All of the passengers are fanning themselves. Suddenly the captain turns on the air and informs us that we might be deplaning shortly and staying the night in Minneapolis—all three hundred of us. After waiting an additional thirty minutes, we are told that we will have to rebook our flight and find a hotel for the night. The ticket agents are standing by to assist us. Ugh. This type of flying is very rough on fibromyalgics. The longer we sit in one position, the stiffer we become—even those of us who are doing well reversing and recovering on Guaifenesin!

I am thankful that I packed my food wisely. It helps me stay clear-headed and powers me through.

Sam has been awaiting our arrival all night. He is excited about our plans for tomorrow. It seems we won't be able to get a flight out of Minnesota until 7:15 Sunday evening, which includes being rerouted back to Michigan and then to LAX. I begin to feel nauseated. You have got to be kidding me!

Michelle remains calm. She is my personal travel agent and informs me that this is *not* going to be our case. We are going to fly directly to LAX in the morning. Something is going to open up for us from the three overbooked flights that are leaving. She assures me that we will be on one of them. I am not to worry.

It is midnight before we go to bed. I am exhausted, yet my body is wired. Yes, very typical for one with fibromyalgia. Since Alexander's birth, I was diagnosed as also having sleep apnea. This was an eye-opener for me because I had related my chronic fatigue to the fact that I was a first time mother who also has fibromyalgia and chronic fatigue syndrome. I now use a CPAP (continuous positive airway pressure) machine every night— a ventilation device that blows a gentle stream of air into the nose during sleep to keep the airway open. It was my first time flying with my CPAP machine, and I am very thankful that I purchased a carry-on with wheels, because we walked nearly ten thousand steps today!

Thank God and the universe for cell phones and Michelle! A great travel tip from my sister—while you are waiting in line for the ticket agent to rebook your flight, call the airline on your cell. Many times, the telephone agent can pull up and find other available flights. It's also wise to call more than once. It seems different agents can offer different flights as things open up, with last-minute cancellations and passengers missing their connectors.

Michelle gets us an earlier flight this way; however, it is not a direct flight to LAX. It is still going to Detroit first but leaving earlier in the day for California. Michelle says not to worry—that we will call first thing in the morning from our hotel and then speak with a few ticket agents once we arrive at the airport. We will be on a direct flight to L.A.!

Sunday, June 8, 2008, Minneapolis, Minnesota *and* Los Angeles, CA—Success! After about six tries by phone and in person, we find two seats on a direct flight to California. We were prepared to fly stand-by, but miraculously two seats opened up.

It is 11 AM California time as we land. Our next adventure is to locate our luggage and catch the shuttle that will take us to the car-rental agency. Our luggage has not arrived yet.

Once our luggage arrives, we pick up the rental car, and Michelle drives us to the hotel. Luckily we brought her GPS. I call Sam and explain the situation. He is thrilled that we are here. Needless to say, Mippy and I are exhausted. We decide to go directly to see Sam; otherwise we fear we won't have time. Our doctor appointment is at 8:30 Monday morning, and we leave to go back to Michigan the following morning. Our time here is short. This is my first time away from Alexander.

We meet up with Sam and his son Howard and spend the evening with them. Sam looks wonderful—not a day older than when I last saw him eight years ago. We decide then and there that Michelle and I will be returning next June for another visit with Dr. St. Amand. Hopefully we will be able to convince my mom to come, too.

## Meeting R. Paul St. Amand, MD

Monday, June 9, 2008, Marina del Rey, CA—I am in his office. This is the moment. This is my time. Five years in the making. I am finally here! I feel like I am meeting a rock star. Dr. St. Amand is exactly as others have described him: kind, caring, patient, funny, relaxed, extremely knowledgeable, and incredibly young-looking and fit for his eighty-one years. I thank him profusely for all that he has done—for helping so many and for being brave and having the courage to write the book with Claudia. By the way, I can't wait to see Claudia again. She is my hero. I had met her one other time when she was in Michigan giving a seminar about a year ago.

I am trying hard to stay in the present moment, but I am anxious to see what Dr. St. Amand finds when he maps me, since I was off of the Guai for seven months last year for pregnancy.

After I answer an assessment of symptomatic questions, I am mapped. My map shows that I am clearing. I might want to raise my dose by 300 mg if it is tolerable. I could cycle faster. I am a low-dose fast responder, which means that I cycle constantly.

I have been on three different types of Guaifenesin in five years. Dr. St. Amand has learned that one of them seems to leach its 100 mg fast-acting white side of the pill into its 500 mg long-acting side, making the long-acting less effective for those of us with fibromyalgia. This medication still does the job but takes longer. He surmises that I have lost eighteen months in the process of my six months on this pill. I find this fascinating, as the world of medicine is always evolving and ever-changing.

I have a laundry list of questions for Dr. St. Amand, my own and ones that I have gathered from support-group members back home. They are as follows:

**Q: What's the best Guaifenesin?**
A: We have had the best luck with the Marina del Rey compounded Guai.

**Q: What other supplements have you found work for migraine headaches?**
A: CoQ10 150 mg has worked for others. The HG diet also helps with migraine headaches if they are blood-sugar related.

**Q: My light sensitivity—do you think that this symptom is my fibromyalgia?**
A: Don't know. It is difficult to discern. If it waxes and wanes and seems to cycle, then it is the excess phosphate in your brain. They can do this. Also, the spasm in the muscles on the left side of your neck presses on the nerves that run behind the eyes.

**Q: Can Guai make your liver enzymes elevate or your liver feel enlarged?**
A: No. Most likely, that is fat. Lose weight and it should reverse.

**Q: Facial hair, hormones, polycystic ovaries—is there any test I should take for this other than the TSH?**
A: No. Try Aldactone the medication for excess facial hair and the low-carb diet.

**Q: Hearing loss—has anyone lost their hearing with fibromyalgia?**
A: I did when I was thirty-one years old. One day it was suddenly gone. It came back in seven days. It is hard to discern. Usually, if it comes back in several days, then it is the fibromyalgia.

**Q: Weight loss and the HG Strict Diet—my weight loss seems to be stalled on the HG Strict Diet. What can I do?**
A: Make sure that you are only eating the foods listed on the diet. No substitutions at all. Cut the calories as much as possible. Eat as much as you want of the pure meat and vegetables.

**Q: Could my cheese stick be involved?**
A: Yes, they now make those cheese sticks with flour to hold them together, and the flour could be throwing your weight loss off. Switch to slices of natural cheese.

**Q: Has anyone been in remission or cured after pregnancy?**
A: We haven't seen anyone.

**Q: I feel shaky when my blood sugar reads on the glucometer in the nineties or in the low one hundreds. Why is this?**
A: You aren't catching it soon enough with your testing. Your body is trying to repair itself, and it is faster than you!

**Q: How long did it take you to reverse?**
A: About seven years, but that was before we knew what we do now about salicylates.

**Q: Do you still play tennis at eighty-one years old?**
A: Yes, I do, but my tennis partner just had back surgery, and I am waiting for him to recover.

**Q: What got you through your fibro?**
A: I had been on uricosuric drugs for forty-six years prior to Guaifenesin.

**Q: Do you have a quote that you live by?**
A: "You deserve perfect. You have already done your old age [with your fibromyalgia]—now it is time for youthing!"

**Q: What does *perfect* entail?**
A: Preventing yourself from becoming diabetic—and all of its complications—by losing the weight you need to by walking and following the diet, along with reversing on the Guaifenesin.

**Q: My doctor would like to have a satellite clinic in Spring Lake, Michigan. Any thoughts?**
A: He is already doing it. He is diagnosing patients and then sending them to the website to learn about salicylates—sending them to you, actually. I would have to learn more about what he has in mind. He would have to hire you. He can give me a call anytime. It is wonderful what you are doing with your support group. We need more people like the both of you out there.

Now we will have the City of Hope Research on file and in print, and if something happens to me, it is documented and will continue. We have raised over $500,000 with donations like yours coming in from all over the world. We can always use more so we can continue the study.

## Being Diagnosed: My Travel Buddy's Shocking Discovery

It is now my sister's turn to be checked for fibromyalgia by Dr. St. Amand. She has made the journey with me as my travel buddy, to make sure that I find my way around. She is still fully functioning, yet I see myself in her. She is becoming more and more plagued with daily migraines, acid reflux, and chronic fatigue.

As a child, she had horrible growing pains, a very common complaint and symptom of fibromyalgia in children, yet often overlooked. She craves sugar, although she is not very overweight and feels that she does not have fibromyalgia, since her muscles don't hurt her very much.

As she talks to Dr. St. Amand, she realizes that her list of symptoms is very long. However, she still doesn't believe that *this* is fibromyalgia. She is not like me. She has not crashed like I have. She reasons that many people have similar symptoms and that they are normal. So we both eagerly await Dr. St. Amand's mapping of her. She doesn't believe that he will find anything. I am certain he will.

At first, he marks nothing on her map. Then he has her bend her head down and forward as he examines her neck. Within seconds, he marks her map. She has a bump at the top of her neck, the base of her skull—the occipital eye region. Immediately my sister and I lunge forward out of our seats to take a closer look at her map. Her body is peppered with fibromyalgia spots. In fact, she has more than I.

So we both ask why she isn't in pain like I am. Dr. St. Amand tells us that she has a higher pain threshold than I do and that she hasn't "crashed" (become completely disabled) yet with it (like I have) and that her most prevalent symptom besides the migraines is chronic fatigue. Wow! This is exactly what I had suspected, but I was always shot down by my family for mentioning it.

Michelle immediately goes into denial mode. I see it in her face because I know her. She is shocked. She can't believe that she has fibromyalgia/chronic fatigue syndrome—although she is plagued with daily fatigue.

Her reaction is normal. The diagnosis of fibromyalgia/chronic fatigue syndrome is a hard one to swallow. None of us wants to imagine that the life we have now could very soon be the life that we left behind if we don't do something proactive like begin the Guaifenesin Protocol.

Michelle doesn't let on that she is skeptical about her diagnosis. We meet with Claudia next to go over the salicylates. She needs to learn about them so she won't block the Guaifenesin.

I am thrilled to see Claudia again. I feel like I have known her all of my life through all of my e-mail contact on the GuaiGroup. She is energetic, kind, intelligent, and soft-spoken. She has a beautiful, soothing voice. She's also lost a large amount of weight since I last saw her nine months ago at the seminar in Michigan. She has been diligently following the strict diet. She is a true inspiration.

Now back to salicylates and Michelle. Michelle and I view Claudia's large walk-in style closet display case of salicylate-free over-the-counter products. Michelle recognizes many of her own products and realizes that she won't have to change many of them, and that is a relief. She could do this part of the protocol. She could take the Guaifenesin and reverse her lumps and bumps.

I insist that she give it a try. I do not want her to wake up one day bedridden like I was. She is lucky—she has a chance at a normal life. The HG diet is another story, something for her to really ponder. She is not yet ready to give up her sweets.

We both agree to enter ourselves and our parents into the City of Hope DNA Research Study that is currently ongoing. We are to bring four vials home with us and collect saliva samples from each parent and ourselves. If my husband and son want to participate, they can also. For now, it will be the four of us in the study. I have to ask Josh about his and Alexander's part in it today. Our sister Nicole won't be participating, as she has not been officially diagnosed with having fibromyalgia. Although Michelle and I suspect that she has it too. Josh agrees that he and Alexander should participate.

We had a wonderful time in the office today with Claudia, Dr. St. Amand, and his receptionist. It was everything and much more than I hoped it would be. Our next stop is the Marina del Rey Pharmacy. I am curious to see what it looks like after ordering from them for years.

How cute. The pharmacy is just outside and next to the Marina del Rey Medical Center. It looks like a building out of the *Jetsons* cartoon. It is a small circular building with windows all around and blue trim around the top. Inside it looks like a normal pharmacy except for its concave shelves. One wall is dedicated to salicylate-free products, almost as I had imagined. It is actually a bit smaller inside than I had thought it would be. But that is okay. It is still *fantastic* to be here and to experience it all. I stock up on Cluere lip balm and lipstick. Michelle and I both put in our prescriptions for the Marina del Rey Guaifenesin and wait for them to be filled.

<u>Monday June 9, 2008, Marina del Rey, CA—</u>Michelle and I decide that we want to make the most of this L.A. experience. We book a Hollywood bus tour for the entire afternoon. We are to view the Hollywood mansions. It leaves in thirty-five minutes, so we scramble (walk over) to a local restaurant to get some food. I have also packed my nuts and my protein powder water. I rely on them to get me through the day. My body needs

them to keep my blood sugar stabilized. I have learned that if I want to be able to think and put a sentence together and not turn into "psycho kitty" with a major migraine, I need to put my blood sugar first and take the time to plan ahead and pack the foods that nourish my body and best feed my brain.

I order a chicken Caesar salad with a side of olive oil and steamed broccoli. My sister orders a chicken wrap. Within minutes, we are in front of the hotel and greeted by a very energetic tour guide, who asks us where we are from and gives us both a huge hug. He is also originally from Michigan. We ask if we can bring our food on the bus, and he says, "Sure." It's a gorgeous day with a blue sky and a calming breeze.

The tour was nothing like we had expected. We had a good laugh, because the celebrity mansions that we saw were from behind and very far off in the distance. We had our pictures taken with the famous Hollywood sign and then spent some time on Rodeo Drive and the Sunset Strip. All in all, it was a wonderful day. I like California. I am shocked at how normal the homes in Beverly Hills looked. Not the gigantic mansions I had envisioned, but charming.

Back at the hotel, Michelle and I compare our fibromyalgia maps, reflect on our reunion with Sam, and begin to plan our return trip for next June.

# Resources

# Tai Chi Range-of-Motion Exercises

These exercises were devised as a series of warm-up exercises prior to actual tai chi exercises. They are meant to increase range of motion of your joints in a passive and non-traumatic way that can be mastered by just about anyone.

The goal is to focus on staying as loose as possible during each of these techniques. The runner's stretch was added due to the fact that people with tight hamstrings invariably develop buttock and low-back pain. By keeping the hamstrings and calves loose, it diminishes low-back pain. Enjoy these and try to implement them daily into your life. They will serve you well. —Thaddeus P. Srutwa, MD

*Always check with your doctor before beginning any exercise routine.

1. **Head Rolls:** Mouth slightly open, drop head to chest and *slowly* rotate left and right four to five times in each direction. Speed is *not* the goal. If discomfort occurs, go just short of the area of discomfort.
2. **Shoulder Rolls:** Envision large wheels being located on your left and right shoulders. Rotate your shoulders *slowly* forward 16-18 times then backwards the same amount of times.
3. **"Helicopter":** Stand with feet shoulder-width apart. Hang arms *loosely* at your sides. Rotate slowly left and right so that your arms flap around to your back and front, lightly slapping those areas sixteen to eighteen times.
4. **"Over and Under":** Right hand on left shoulder, left hand under right arm. Swing both arms forward, then reverse the sequence, so that left hand is on the right shoulder and the right

arm is under your left arm. Repeat this with a slight slapping of the areas of contact for a total of sixteen to eighteen times total.

5. **"Slap your Shoulders":** Swing both arms over the tops of your shoulders so that you slap your shoulder blades each time sixteen to eighteen times.
6. **"Choir Stance":** Hand in front, clasped over and under. Rotate *slowly* to the left and right in as wide a turn as possible without turning at the waist.
7. **"Hula-Hoop":** Head is level (like on a plumb line). Hands on waist. Rotate pelvis without moving head to the left and right, sixteen to eighteen times.
8. **"Shake Hands":** Arms *loosely* at sides. Shake vigorously till warm and tingling. Usually takes about a minute.
9. **"Shake the Feet":** Same principle as #8. Hold a wall for support, remove shoes, and shake each leg vigorously till warm and tingling.
10. **"Runner's Stretch":** Face wall and place palms against it at shoulder height. Place right foot forward to touch wall and find comfortable location for left foot, about a pace behind you. Try to keep your feet in a parallel line if possible. Lean forward *slowly* and push your chest to the wall. Feel the stretch of your right calf as you do this. Then push yourself away from the wall without moving your legs and feel the right thigh and hamstring area stretch. Reverse the process for the opposite leg.

# Daily Fibro Symptom List

Daily Fibromyalgia Symptom List ✓off

| | 1 | 2 | 3 | 4 | 5 | 6 | 7 | 8 | 9 | 10 | 11 | 12 | 13 | 14 | 15 | 16 | 17 | 18 | 19 | 20 | 21 | 22 | 23 | 24 | 25 | 26 | 27 | 28 | 29 | 30 | 31 |
|---|---|---|---|---|---|---|---|---|---|---|---|---|---|---|---|---|---|---|---|---|---|---|---|---|---|---|---|---|---|---|---|
| Headaches | | | | | | | | | | | | | | | | | | | | | | | | | | | | | | | |
| Sinuses | | | | | | | | | | | | | | | | | | | | | | | | | | | | | | | |
| Eye Pain | | | | | | | | | | | | | | | | | | | | | | | | | | | | | | | |
| Dry Eyes | | | | | | | | | | | | | | | | | | | | | | | | | | | | | | | |
| Burning Eyes | | | | | | | | | | | | | | | | | | | | | | | | | | | | | | | |
| FATIGUE | | | | | | | | | | | | | | | | | | | | | | | | | | | | | | | |
| Fog (Brain) | | | | | | | | | | | | | | | | | | | | | | | | | | | | | | | |
| INSOMNIA | | | | | | | | | | | | | | | | | | | | | | | | | | | | | | | |
| Ringing Ears | | | | | | | | | | | | | | | | | | | | | | | | | | | | | | | |
| Light Sensit | | | | | | | | | | | | | | | | | | | | | | | | | | | | | | | |
| Noise Sensit | | | | | | | | | | | | | | | | | | | | | | | | | | | | | | | |
| Dizziness | | | | | | | | | | | | | | | | | | | | | | | | | | | | | | | |
| Nausea | | | | | | | | | | | | | | | | | | | | | | | | | | | | | | | |
| Neck | | | | | | | | | | | | | | | | | | | | | | | | | | | | | | | |
| Shoulders | | | | | | | | | | | | | | | | | | | | | | | | | | | | | | | |
| Arms | | | | | | | | | | | | | | | | | | | | | | | | | | | | | | | |
| Wrists | | | | | | | | | | | | | | | | | | | | | | | | | | | | | | | |
| Hands/Fingers | | | | | | | | | | | | | | | | | | | | | | | | | | | | | | | |
| ♥ Burn | | | | | | | | | | | | | | | | | | | | | | | | | | | | | | | |
| IBS | | | | | | | | | | | | | | | | | | | | | | | | | | | | | | | |
| Upper Back | | | | | | | | | | | | | | | | | | | | | | | | | | | | | | | |
| Mid Back | | | | | | | | | | | | | | | | | | | | | | | | | | | | | | | |
| Lower Back Buttocks | | | | | | | | | | | | | | | | | | | | | | | | | | | | | | | |
| Knees | | | | | | | | | | | | | | | | | | | | | | | | | | | | | | | |
| Elbow | | | | | | | | | | | | | | | | | | | | | | | | | | | | | | | |
| Legs | | | | | | | | | | | | | | | | | | | | | | | | | | | | | | | |
| Feet/Toes | | | | | | | | | | | | | | | | | | | | | | | | | | | | | | | |
| Rash | | | | | | | | | | | | | | | | | | | | | | | | | | | | | | | |
| Burning Bladder | | | | | | | | | | | | | | | | | | | | | | | | | | | | | | | |
| Diet cheat | | | | | | | | | | | | | | | | | | | | | | | | | | | | | | | |
| Numbness | | | | | | | | | | | | | | | | | | | | | | | | | | | | | | | |

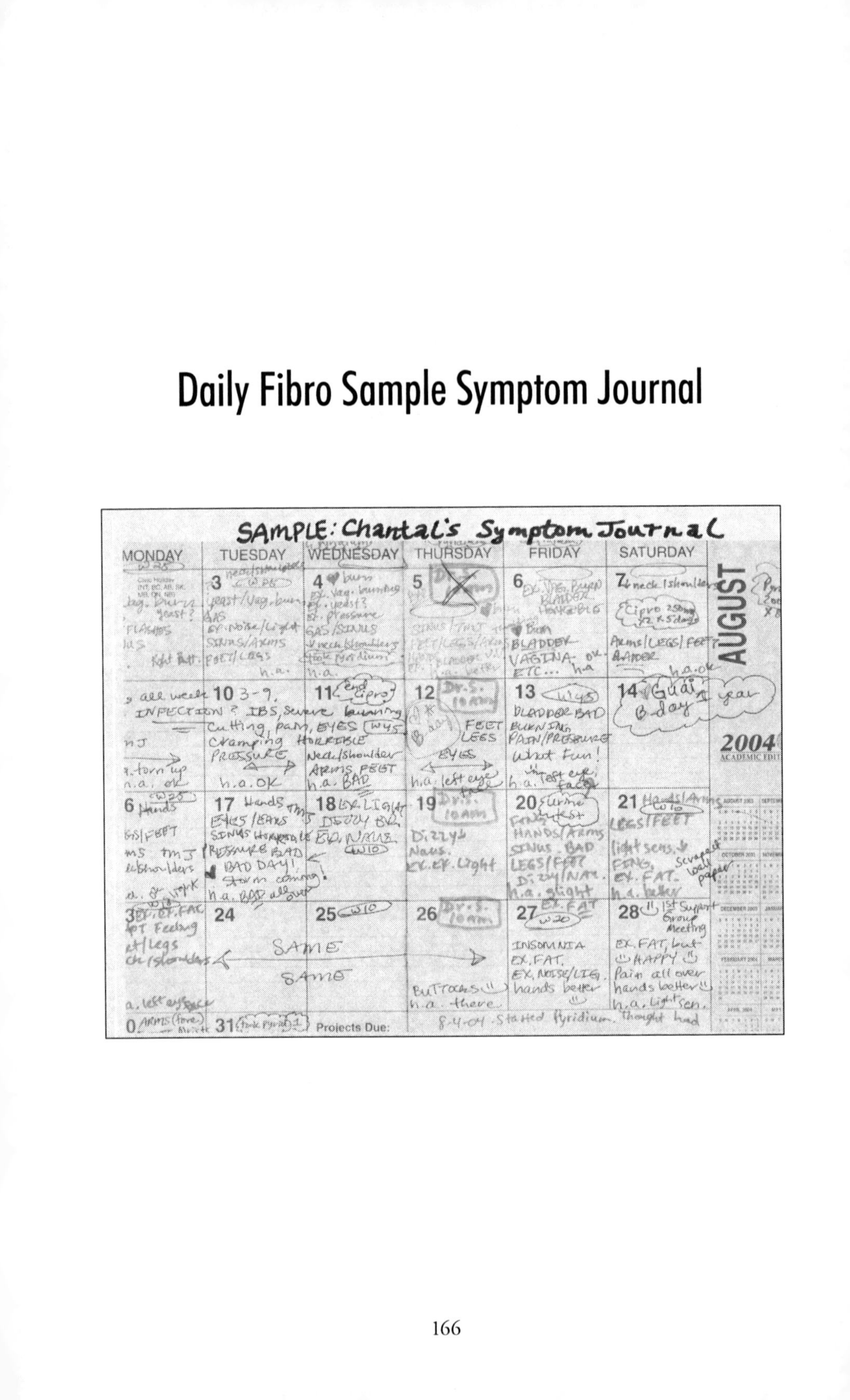

# Daily Fibro Sample Symptom Journal

SAMPLE: Chantal's Symptom Journal

# Chantal's Map August 2007

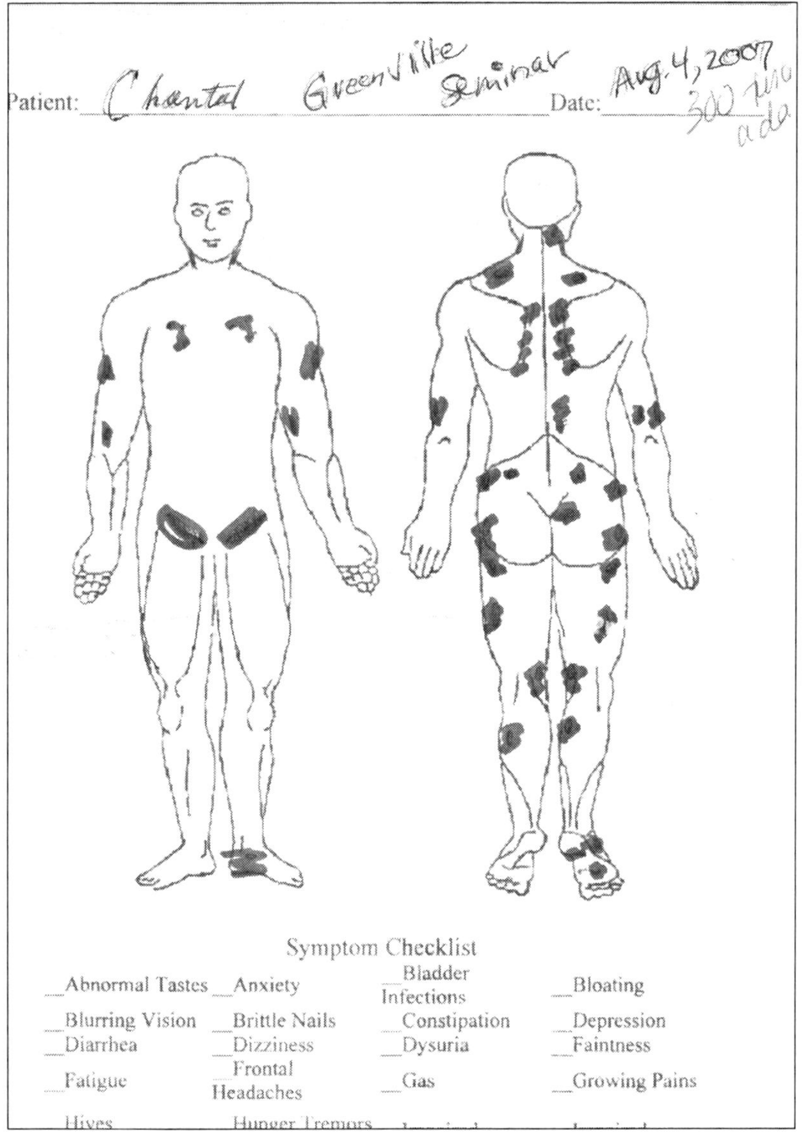

Patient: Chantal Greenville Seminar Date: Aug. 4, 2007 300 [illegible]

Symptom Checklist

| | | | |
|---|---|---|---|
| __Abnormal Tastes | __Anxiety | __Bladder Infections | __Bloating |
| __Blurring Vision | __Brittle Nails | __Constipation | __Depression |
| __Diarrhea | __Dizziness | __Dysuria | __Faintness |
| __Fatigue | __Frontal Headaches | __Gas | __Growing Pains |
| __Hives | __Hunger Tremors | | |

# Baby Registry Must-Haves for the Fibromyalgic Mother-to-Be:

*On a budget*—www.craigslist.org *sells gently used baby gear;* www.freecycle.org *lists free items ready to be discarded*

(Copy this list, take it with you, and use it as your guide.)

Remember to register for larger sizes too. This will make changes easier on your fibromyalgic fingers, hands, and wrists. Also, babies grow quickly, and you might end up with a nine-pound-plus baby like I did who was wearing a size twelve months at six months!

**Bolded items are my "Best Baby Invention" must-haves, and I have rated my top ten for you.**

- **6–8 Sleepsacks by Halo Innnovations.** (These are usually part of the Layette, but not always. They are a must in the prevention of SIDS. (My #1 Best Baby Invention!) Available at *www.target.com* or *www.walmart.com.* Also available in larger sizes for toddlers too: Halo Big Kids.
- **2–4 Snack Catchers** A special cup with a toddler-friendly lid and handles used for holding Cheerios and snacks without spilling or a parent's help. Available online at Amazon.com (My other #1 Best Baby Invention.)
- **Graco Snugride Car Seat Travel System or the like.** (Make sure that you buy the car seat that snaps into the base and the stroller that goes with the car seat. The stroller will double as a high chair in restaurants when baby gets older and can

sit up. If buying used, check expiration dates. Regulations change and car seats expire every six years.) (My #2 Best Baby Invention.)

- **Crib Tent** if you have cats for crib and playard. (My #3 Best Baby Invention.) Available online at *www.walmart.com.*
- **Graco Pack N Play**—Great for travel and Grandma's house. Can be used as both a changing station and a bassinet. (My #4 Best Baby Invention.)
- **Breathable Bumper**—instead of traditional bumpers. This bumper will grow with your baby when he or she starts to flip over onto his or her tummy, and you won't have to worry about baby getting caught under it. (My other #4 Best Baby Invention.)
- **Diaper Champ** (My #5 Best Baby Invention.)
- **2–4 Munchkin Food Bags** (My # 6 Best Baby Invention.)
- **Playtex Insulator Sippy Cup** After trying several. This cup holds up when thrown and doesn't leak. (My # 7 Best Baby Invention.)
- **2-Sassy Teether Car Keys** (My # 8 Best Baby Invention.)
- **2–4 Sassy Mirrors** for the crib and the changing stations (Best Baby Invention.)
- **Appliance "Locks" Self-Adhesive Locks** that won't damage paint and can be used in place of other cabinet and drawer locks. (My # 9 Best Baby Invention.) Available at Target.
- **Monkey Backpack Harness** (My #10 Best Baby Invention.) Available at Target.
- **The First Years Night and Day Bottle Warmer** Used for heating up bottles and jars of baby food. Includes a cooler. (Best Baby Invention.)
- Straps for attaching bookshelves and other large furniture to the walls. (Best Baby Invention.)
- **Electrical Outlet Covers (Switch Plates)** that move. (Best Baby Invention.)
- **2–4 Sippy Cup Leashes** available online at Amazon.com (Best Baby Invention.)
- **Exersaucer** for when baby is around 6 months. (Best Baby Invention.)
- **Diaper Backpack Land's End or Dad's Gear** (Best Baby Invention.)

- Crib that meets today's safety standards.
- 4–6 crib sheets.
- Bassinet—on a budget, the Pack N Play is sufficient until baby reaches recommended weight.
- Changing station or two. (Make sure that they have drawers instead of shelves, as baby will pull everything off of the shelves when he or she learns to walk. And you will be out buying another station. Also, check the weight limit of the changing table. Some tables are made to hold only twenty to twenty-three pounds.) On a budget, the Pack N Play is sufficient until weight requirement is met.
- Nightlights for bathroom, hallway, nursery.
- Fifteen-watt baby lamp for nighttime changes that won't wake baby.
- Bouncer.
- Swing, the Fisher-Price Take-Along Swing is wonderful.
- 2–4 Layette sets—(The layette set usually includes a onesie, a hat, a sleeper, and a sleep sack. Sometimes it will include a bib and booties.)
- 4 packages of onesies—any brand. All sizes. (I prefer Gerber, as they are stretchy, easy to put on with my fibromyalgic hands, and they grow well with baby.)
- 6–8 receiving blankets.
- Package of newborn diapers.
- 10 sleepers—zippered are best for fibromyalgic hands.
- 2 packages of washcloths.
- Gerber baby feeding spoons.
- Madela Hand-held Breast Pump Starter Kit (I also purchased the Madela Electric Pump.)
- Lanolin—if breastfeeding.
- Soothies for breastfeeding.

# Tips on What to Pack for the Hospital for the Fibromyalgic Mother-to-Be

Keep in mind when packing for the hospital that they will provide certain items for you, such as sanitary napkins and baby supplies, so you don't need to overpack. I overpacked!

Make sure that you pack the normal comfort measures that you use on a daily basis at home, such as heating pad, ice packs, or special pillow. I packed protein powder and nuts for a protein boost for *after* the baby was born.

Most hospitals won't allow you to eat during labor or delivery. I had been worried about my hypoglycemia, but my body seemed to reset itself after about six hours of not eating.

If you use a bite splint, don't be shy about wearing it during your hospital stay, childbirth, and delivery. It may save you TMJ and headache pain.

If you are noise-sensitive, pack earplugs. If you are light-sensitive, like I am, pack your sunglasses. I wore mine for my whole hospital stay, including during my labor and delivery.

If you are hypoglycemic, like I am, pack some protein powder to mix with water for after delivery. You most likely will be given only ice chips while in labor. Don't worry. I was afraid that I was going to bottom out blood sugar-wise while giving birth, but I didn't. Once the baby was born and I was given the all-clear to order some food, I ordered myself a steak and green beans. My mom and my sister just laughed at me. After twelve hours of labor and two and a half hours of hard pushing, I knew that I needed the protein.

# Hospital Packing List for the Fibromyalgic Mother-to-Be

## What to Pack for Mom:

- Any prescription drugs that you take; must notify nurses of any meds you bring
- Pillow and brightly colored pillowcase
- Nightgown and robe
- Going-home clothes, clothes your wore at around six months pregnant
- Toothbrush
- Toothpaste
- Lotion
- Hairbrush
- Deodorant
- Eye drops
- Make-up, if needed
- Portable stereo and music or iPod
- Glasses and/or contact lenses and supplies
- Bite splint
- Earplugs
- Sunglasses, if needed
- Sugar-free hard candy to suck after delivery and for hubby or partner
- Small cooler with cheese sticks and protein powder
- Bottled water to mix protein powder in
- Small funnel to put protein powder into bottle

## What to Pack for Baby:

- Car seat already installed
- Newborn outfit for hospital picture
- Newborn going-home outfit
- 2 receiving blankets
- 2 onesies
- 4 newborn diapers
- Small package of wipes

## What to Pack for Husband or Partner:

- Change of clothes
- Toothbrush
- Toothpaste
- Deodorant
- Mouthwash
- Snacks: nuts, crackers, cheese, hard candy

# Notes


## Chapter 1

Hay, Louise. *You Can Heal Your Life* [Sound recording]. Santa Monica: Hay House, 1988.

## Chapter 3

Kabat-Zinn, Jon, PhD. *Wherever You Go, There You Are* [Audiobook]. New York: Audio Renaissance, 2001.

Miller, Emmett, MD. *The 10-Minute Stress Manager* [Audiobook]. Carlsbad: Hay House Audio Books, 2005.

Myss, Caroline. *Anatomy of the Spirit: The Seven Stages of Power and Healing.* Three Rivers Press, 1997.

Myss, Caroline. *Sacred Contracts: Awakening Your Divine Potential* [Audiobook]. Boulder: Sounds True, 2001.

Orloff, Judith, MD. *Second Sight* [Audio Cassette, abridged edition]. Audio Literature, 1997.

Orloff, Judith, MD. *Positive Energy: 10 Extraordinary Prescriptions for Transforming Fatigue, Stress, and Fear into Vibrance, Strength, and Love* [Audio Cassette, abridged edition]. New York: Random House Audio, 2004.

## Chapter 4

Starlanyl, Devin. *The Fibromyalgia Advocate.* (Berkeley: New Harbinger Publications, Inc., 1999).

## Chapter 5

Lipton, Bruce, PhD. *The Biology of Belief: Unleashing the Power of Consciousness, Matter, and Miracles* (Santa Rosa: Mountain of Love/Elite Books, 2005) 123-144.

## Chapter 6

*Love Chords: Classical Music to Enrich the Bond with Your Unborn Child* [Audio CD]. Burlington: Children's Book Store Distribution, 1998.

Mazel, Sharon and Murkoff, Heidi.*What to Expect When You're Expecting* (New York: Workman Publishing Company; 4 edition, 2008).

Murkoff, Heidi and Mazel, Sharon. *What to Expect: Eating Well When You're Expecting* (New York: Workman Publishing Company; 1 edition, 2005).

Marek, Claudia Craig. *The First Year: Fibromyalgia: A Patient-Expert Walks You Through Everything You Need to Learn and Do* (New York: Da Capo Press; First edition, 2003).

CPSIA information can be obtained at www.ICGtesting.com
Printed in the USA
BVOW07*1835170614

356636BV00001B/6/P